David Lester

The "I" of the Storm: Understanding the Suicidal Mind

David Lester

The "I" of the Storm

Understanding the Suicidal Mind

Managing Editor: Aneta Przepiórka

DE GRUYTER
OPEN

Published by De Gruyter Open Ltd, Warsaw/Berlin

ISBN: 978-3-11-037481-0
e-ISBN: 978-3-11-037482-7

Bibliographic information published by the Deutsche Nationalbibliothek
The Deutsche Nationalbibliothek lists this publication in the Deutsche Nationalbibliografie; detailed bibliographic data are available in the Internet at http://dnb.dnb.de.

Managing Editor: Aneta Przepiórka

www.degruyteropen.com

Cover illustration: © ThinkStock/andreusK

Contents

Preface

I have published a lot on suicide – some say much too much! I have written four editions of a book call *Why People Kill Themselves* which summarize one hundred years of suicide research from 1897 to 1997, although it has been pointed out that none of them explain why people kill themselves! However, I realized a few years ago that I had no idea why people die by suicide. I have sat around the backyard pool of a colleague of mine who is also a suicidologist, and we agree that neither of us has any idea why people kill themselves. I decided, therefore, that, if I could understand why just one person chose to die by suicide, I could continue doing my research and publishing my articles and books which throw little light on the answer to the question. This book documents my attempt to understand that one person.

Why can't we explain why people choose suicide? We know many, many risk factors and warning signs that predict suicide. Among the risk factors are neurophysiological (e.g., serotonin levels), psychiatric (e.g., diagnosis), intrapsychic (e.g., emotional dysregulation), experiential (e.g., stressful life events), interpersonal (e.g., broken relationships), and societal (e.g., oppression and discrimination) variables. Among the possible warning signs are those proposed by the American Association of Suicidology (www.suicidology.org), summarized by the mnemonic IS PATH WARM (Suicidal Ideation, Substance abuse, Purposelessness, Anger, Trapped, Hopelessness, Withdrawing, Anxiety, Recklessness, and Mood change).

But there is no necessary or sufficient cause for suicide. The reason for this, of course, is that suicide is so rare. Some 35,000 people will kill thsemlves in the United States this year, but picking those 35,000 out from 313,000,000 Americans is extremely difficult, if not impossible. Even if we had a good screening instrument, the problem of false positives would ruin our chances of identifying and preventing those suicides.

Let us assume we have a population of 10,000 patients in a hospital or inmates in a prison with a suicide rate of 20 per 100,000 per year. Let us assume that our screening instrument is 75% accurate. There will be two suicides next year, but our screening instrument will identify 2,500 possible suicides. If the screening instrument is 90% accurate, it will identify 1,000 possible suicides; if it is 95% accurate (much more accurate than any existing screening instrument) it will identify 500 possible suicides. That is far too many false positives for an institution to cope with. The *Journal of the American Medical Association* published my humorous letter on this issue in 1974.

> ……This suggests that we could prevent suicide more easily if it were more common, in which case the proportion of false positives would be much lower
>
> This in turn suggests that, in order to prevent suicide more effectively, we must increase the suicide rate. Only then will be able to reduce the suicide rate! (Lester, 1974, p. 26-27)

Rather than *explaining suicide* (looking for causes), perhaps we can *understand suicide*, at least in one individual, a phenomenological approach. I began that task by reading a biography of a famous suicide because biographies of famous individuals contain a wealth of detail about every aspect of their lives. I began with Ernest Hemingway, and I felt that I understood why he killed himself when he did and in the way that he did. However, as far as suicidology is concerned, I am an obsessive-compulsive. I have now read over one hundred biographies of famous suicides (famous enough to have a biography written). You can find some of my essays on them on my website (www.drdavidlester.net).

Serendipitously, I was given the diary of a suicide. An undergraduate student of mine possessed the diary of her sister who killed herself and asked me whether I would be interested in it. I said yes, and I obtained her permission to edit a book on the diary. I asked my colleagues in the field to contribute chapters, resulting in *Katie's Diary: Unlocking the Mystery of a Suicide* (Lester, 2004b).

Since then I have collected nine diaries from suicides (and two from attempted suicides). I have also studied the poems of those who chose suicide (both famous poets and unpublished poets), the letters written by suicides, and one tape recording of a young man who killed himself just an hour or so after he recorded the tape. This book will tell you what I have learned from my studies of these materials. But I should warn you. It may not be possible to generalize from one individual to another. If we obtain some insights into the mind of one suicidal individual, this may not help us understand another suicidal individual. But it might, and certainly the technique may illustrate one pathway to understanding.

1 The Study of Personal Documents by Those Who Died by Suicide

There is a long history of using written material to illustrate and sometimes test psychological theories of suicide (Lester 1987), for example, by using the content of suicide notes (Leenaars 1988). Occasionally, suicides (such as Sylvia Plath) leave a book or poem describing their behavior, and this kind of material may be of use in exploring the unconscious psychodynamics of the suicidal act. This chapter will briefly review this earlier work.

1.1 Studying Suicide through Literature

1.1.1 Understanding Suicide

Faber (1970) has provided several examples of how an examination of suicide in literary characters can throw light on our understanding of suicide. In doing this, Faber explicitly states that he views literary suicides as case studies (although he places the words in quotes) which may serve as archetypes of suicidal behavior and which may provide insights into suicidal behavior. He states that he is not interested in how the suicides further the literary aims or "esthetic contraptions" of the authors, their esthetic implications or how they might throw light on the attitudes toward suicide of the society in which the play was written.

In Faber's analyses of the suicide of Haemon in Sophocles' *Antigone* and the self-blinding of Oedipus in his *Oedipus The King*, Faber provides useful insights into the unconscious motivation for suicide, since Sophocles appears to have anticipated Freud's insights by some two thousand years. However, Freud's theory could just as easily have been illustrated with modern cases. On the other hand, many of the suicides in the plays of Euripides are altruistic suicides, and altruistic suicide is rare in modern times. Few case studies appear in print, and many suicidologists have suggested removing altruistic and fatalistic suicide from Durkheim's (1897) theory since these types of suicide are so rare in modern society (Johnson 1965).

The suicide of Alcestis, Queen of Thessaly, illustrates some of the possible unconscious psychodynamics of voluntary altruistic suicide. Apollo learns that Alcestis's husband, Admetus, is to die prematurely and makes a deal with the Fates to spare his life. The Fates demand another death in Admetus's place, and only his wife, Alcestis, volunteers to die in his place.

The central theme in the play appears not to be that Alcestis has offered to die in place of her husband, but that her husband has accepted her offer! After Alcestis realizes that her husband is going to accept her offer, she is filled with resentment toward him. She acts so as to induce guilt in him in order to punish him for accepting her offer. However, her aggression is expressed in part consciously and in part unconsciously.

On the day of her death, Alcestis does not emphasize the voluntary nature of her death. She speaks of herself as one who is about to be destroyed, implying that Admetus should have protected her from this destruction. She hints of betrayal and abandonment, focusing for example on her soon-to-be-motherless children. She expresses the hope that her daughter will marry a noble husband, implying that her own husband is not so noble. In Admetus's presence, Alcestis breaks down and weeps, whereas with others she is more controlled. As soon as Admetus begins to experience the guilt and to suffer, Alcestis recovers her composure rapidly. She then extracts a promise from Admetus that he will not remarry, so that he will be less likely to forget Alcestis and her sacrifice.

Faber notes that Admetus is very dependent upon his wife, and it is this dependence that leads him in part to ask for and accept her sacrifice. However, his dependency on Alcestis makes her loss unbearable. He ends up begging her not to abandon him. We have, therefore, a relationship between a dependent person with few inner resources and a self-sacrificing person who resents being involved with a man who needs her in an infantile way, as an object. Admetus uses Alcestis's sacrifice to stop living rather than anticipating the construction of a new life without her.

So, a clinical hypothesis generated by Faber's analysis is that voluntary altruistic suicides think that they are victims; in contrast, obligatory altruistic suicides tend to protect their egos by transforming the will of others into their own will, that is, they see themselves as martyrs. I doubt that this hypothesis could have been formulated using cases of suicidal behavior found among the clinical material in the files of psychiatric hospitals or psychotherapists' offices.

1.1.2 Understanding a Culture

Suicides in literature have also been used to study a culture. Lester (1972) examined the suicides which occurred in the plays of the Norwegian Henrik Ibsen (1828-1906) to see if they conformed to the patterns described by Hendin (1964) for suicides in Norway, Sweden or Denmark. Hendin used his clinical judgment to argue that suicide in Sweden was usually the result of failure to achieve a high level of performance, suicide in Denmark was the result of the loss of significant others, and suicide in Norway was the result either of loss of a significant other upon whom the suicide was dependent or the result of guilt over transgressions.

Apart from a brief mention in *Cataline* of the suicide of a woman after rape, there are seven suicidal deaths in Ibsen's plays, five victim-precipitated homicides and two equivocal deaths. In general, Lester found that the suicides had suffered from dependency loss whereas the victim-precipitated murders were experiencing guilt over transgressions. The suicides also appeared to be motivated by the desire to preserve or restore an ideal self-image.

For example, in *The Wild Duck*, Hedvig is very attached to her parents, especially her father. Because of her poor eyesight, she does not go to school and has no friends her own age. Hedvig's suicide occurs after her father realizes that she is not his daughter, considers leaving home, and verbally rejects her. Hedvig shoots herself shortly after her father tells her to go away and not to come near him. Her suicide is clearly provoked by the rejection from her father. It would seem to be a dependency-loss suicide, which fits Hendin's description of Norwegian suicides.[1]

1.1.3 Understanding a Suicidal Writer

There are several suicidal writers whose fiction appears to be somewhat autobiographical which, therefore, provides us with some insights into their unconscious psychodynamics which increases our understanding of them, authors such as Ernest Hemingway and Cesare Pavese. Sylvia Plath (1981, pp. 183-184) wrote a single poem (*Daddy*) in the months prior to her suicide which provides a startling insight into the psychodynamics of her suicide.

In *Daddy*, Plath casts herself as a Jew in a concentration camp versus her father as a Panzer man and as a devil who bit her heart in two. She says that she has always been scared of him, and she calls him a bastard. Yet she says that her suicide attempt at age twenty was an attempt to be reunited with him. She then made of model of her father and married him, but she calls this person a vampire who drank her blood for seven years. Indeed, her marriage to the British poet, Ted Hughes, lasted about seven years. At the end of her poem, she tells her father that he can lie back now, perhaps because, as she says a few lines earlier, that she is finally through, presumably with life, and is now coming back to him

The Oedipal theme in the poem is clear. The motivation for her first suicide attempt was to be reunited with the father who died when she was eight (though the poem says ten). And, in case he is jealous of her marriage to Ted Hughes (why else is Daddy sitting up in his grave), she is now finally through and, presumably, going to be reunited with Daddy for sure this time (and so he can lie back down to await her).

In addition, there are other elements in the poem. The ambivalence toward her father is evident throughout the poem, but most exquisitely expressed in the final line where she writes, "Daddy, daddy, you bastard...," a juxtaposition of affection (daddy) and anger (you bastard). Plath also says that, "If I've killed one man, I've killed two." Who are these two? Daddy and her husband? Plath's father died of natural causes

1 Interestingly, Ibsen considered moving to Denmark, but never did so. Furthermore, according to Meyer (1971), Ibsen did contemplate suicide during one stressful period in his life.

when she was eight, but perhaps Sylvia had wished his death when she was angry at him and believes, magically, that her death wish for him contributed to his death, a common belief in children. Or perhaps she feels guilty over other of her actions toward her father before he died? But then, how did she kill her husband? Perhaps psychologically, as her stature as a poet grew to equal, and perhaps surpass, his? There is an interesting feature to this poem in that Plath uses the word "black" six times, a frequency much higher than in her first book of poems (Lester 1989a). According to Piotrowski's (1974) method for interpreting the Rorschach ink-blot test, the use of dark shading predicts a tendency to act-out, rather than quieten down, when anxious or under stress.[2]

1.2 Does Creative Writing Harm Suicidal People?

Is writing therapeutic for creative writers or it is a stressor which contributes to their psychological disturbance? Silverman and Will (1986) analyzed the life and suicide of Sylvia Plath and concluded that, although she tried to control her suicidal impulses by means of her poetry, she failed in this endeavor. Silverman and Will argued that poetry is successful when it bridges the inner worlds of the creative person and the audience. (Presumably they mean critically successful, for even poor poetry can serve a useful psychological function for the writer, even if it is merely cathartic.) To be successful, poetry must first achieve a balance between the writer's use of the audience to serve his or her own narcissistic needs (a type of exhibitionism) and the desire to give others a way of structuring the terrors and anxieties that afflict us all (a homonomous desire on the part of the writer to use a term coined by Andras Angyal [1965]).

The writer must also achieve a balance between the potentially destructive conscious and unconscious forces motivating the writing and the constructive desires to harness these forces for the purpose of writing creatively. Related to this, the writer must balance primary and secondary process mechanisms. The writer must also compromise between the fantasy permissible in writing and the acceptance of reality necessary for successful living.

When they applied their ideas to Sylvia Plath, Silverman and Will asserted that the successful creative process is successful only when the unconscious forces in the writer operate silently and remain hidden from view. This assertion represents a rather traditional view of creative writing. It would seem to express a preference on the part of Silverman and Will for a particular type of literature rather than expressing a universal truth. For example, the unconscious forces motivating Ernest Hemingway may be under control in his writing, but they are certainly not hidden. More pertinently,

2 Lester (1991c) noted a similar tendency in the poems of Anne Sexton, who also died by suicide.

the confessional style of poetry developed by W. D. Snodgrass and Robert Lowell and pursued by Anne Sexton is in direct opposition to Silverman and Will's view.

Silverman and Will saw the transitional period in Plath's poetry as being her final years in the United States. Plath may have had her confidence undermined by the frequent rejections that writers must endure so that she changed her style. In her new style, she revealed her deepest feelings in her poems, using her experiences to create the poem rather than to simply transform it. Silverman and Will noted that she described her early poems as "proper in shape and number and every part" but not alive. Her poems moved from being a reordering and reshaping of experience with a poetic purpose toward becoming expressions of herself. She identified with her poems, which made their rejection even more painful, and Silverman and Will labeled this change as a "narcissistic regression."

The causal sequence which Silverman and Will proposed for Plath has no evidence for or against it. It is simply one reading of Plath's life. Other, equally plausible, alternative paths can be proposed. For example, it is quite likely that Plath's participation, along with Anne Sexton with whom she became very close, in a poetry workshop run by Robert Lowell had a major impact on her writing style. Several members of his workshop adopted a more self-revealing content for their poems, and two received Pulitzer prizes for their work (Lowell and Sexton).

Furthermore, Plath, as she herself clearly recognized, was prone to recurring depressions. In all probability, Plath had an affective disorder, possibly bipolar, and her depressions were likely to reoccur periodically. It is evident from the severity of her depression in 1953 which led to a very serious suicide attempt that she would likely become suicidal again with each new depression (much as Virginia Woolf had).

What is interesting is that, whereas in the early 1950s, her writing may not have helped her cope with the stressors, external and intrapsychic, with which she was confronted, in the later 1950s her switch to a more revealing and personalized style of writing may have helped her survive. Silverman and Will claimed that her writing failed to prevent her suicide. Perhaps it may have postponed her suicide?

In the months prior to her suicide, Plath wrote feverishly, sometimes producing several poems in one day. (This feverish activity in the months prior to a suicide was apparent also in Anne Sexton's life.) What would Silverman and Will suggest as a more appropriate strategy for a person confronting intrapsychic turmoil who is not under professional care? It is very likely that the writing helped Plath control her inner turmoil, and some commentators think that the poems she produced were among her finest.

In seeking to formulate a *general* hypothesis about the role of writing for the depressed and distressed person, it is obviously important to discuss more than one case. In the present context, the life and suicide of the poet Anne Sexton is relevant. Lester and Terry (1992) argued that writing poetry can be useful with suicidal clients. Writing poems *per se* may not be helpful to the client, but the revision of the initial drafts of poems may be therapeutically useful. Revising poems may serve a similar function for clients as the journal assignments devised by cognitive therapists by giving the clients intellectual control over their emotions and distance from the traumatic memories. Sexton revised her poems extensively and, in the process of revision, had to concentrate on form rather than content. This allows for both the action that therapists deem to be therapeutic and the distancing of the self from one's problems. Because Sexton ultimately chose the moment of her death, one should not discount the therapeutic help her writing afforded her.

Anne Sexton illustrates the dialectic in poetry as therapy, between expression and catharsis on the one hand and cognitive control on the other. Sexton, as long as she was able to stay psychiatrically stable, was able to apply the craft of poetry to her creative productions. Both Sexton and Martin Orne, her first therapist, believed that her poetry had helped her recover. Only toward the end of her life, as her ability to craft her poems declined, so did her mental stability dissipate.

Interestingly, both Plath and Sexton showed manic trends prior to their suicides, writing poems furiously, poems with more emotional expression and less poetic crafting. Rather than arguing that writing poetry contributed in part to their suicides, it makes much more sense to say that, in their final breakdowns, poetry was no longer able to help them deal with the intrapsychic forces driving them as it had in the past. As their inner turmoil increased, both wrote feverishly, almost like a safety valve letting out the steam under pressure in a boiler, but to no avail since the pressure was building up faster than they could release it.

But this final failure of the craft of poetry to keep Sylvia Plath and Anne Sexton alive does not, as Silverman and Will argued, signify total failure. Both were outstanding poets and functioned quite well given their probable affective disorders. I would argue that the craft of poetry kept both poets alive for many years after their self-destructive impulses first manifested themselves and so signifies success.[3]

1.2.1 The Use of Personal Documents

The study of personal documents in psychology also has a long history, but it received strong support from Gordon Allport who urged such study in general (Allport, 1942) and who provided many illustrations. For example, Allport (1965) reprinted a series of letters from a woman, whom he named Jenny, to a friend in order to see whether they could "explain" Jenny.

3 It should be noted in passing that creative writing has been found to be strongly associated with both affective disorder (Andreasen, 1987; Holden, 1987) and with alcohol abuse (Goodwin, 1988), and these disorders may adversely affect the psychological health of writers.

> Why does an intelligent lady behave so persistently in a self-defeating manner? When and how might she have averted the tragedy of her life?.....Was the root of her trouble some wholly unconscious mechanism? (Allport, 1965, p. viii)

In the book, Allport used the letters to provide psychodynamic, existential, learning and trait descriptions of Jenny.

The use of personal documents in the study of suicide has played a prominent role because there is so little information available on individual suicides. The majority of suicides leave no clinical records and, when they do, perhaps as a result of being in psychotherapy or being hospitalized in a psychiatric facility, the records are not standardized. As a result, it is difficult to collect comparable data or psychological test scores from a sample of such suicides.

However, a good proportion of suicides, perhaps as many as 40 percent, do leave suicide notes. In the 1950s, Edwin Shneidman and Norman Farberow (1957b) published their first study of a sample of suicide notes that they found in the files of the Los Angeles medical examiner's office, and the study of suicide notes is the focus of Part 2 of this book.

1.3 The Use of Diaries

Diaries may provide an excellent way of delving into the psychodynamics of people's lives. Culley (1985) thought that a diary gives shape and meaning to the writer's life, and so a reading of the diary should give us insights into this meaning. Kagle (1979) argued that diaries would be affected by tensions and disequilibria in the life of the writer that need to be resolved. Such diaries may prove to be more of a "royal road to the unconscious" than are dreams. An example of the use of diaries in the exploration of psychodynamics is Brumberg (1997) who studied diaries from young girls to show how a focus on the development of internal character in the late 1800s changed to a focus on the shape and appearance of their bodies in the late 1900s.

Some suicides leave diaries. The most accessible diaries of this kind are those written by famous writers who have killed themselves. The diaries of Sylvia Plath have been published (Plath, 2000) although, unfortunately, her husband, Ted Hughes, destroyed one diary and lost another which, together, cover the last three years of her life. The diaries of Cesare Pavese have also appeared in print (Pavese, 1961). Occasionally, diaries of others, less famous, have appeared in print, such as those of Arthur Inman (1985).

But what of the diaries of ordinary individuals, more representative of the typical suicide, but not sufficiently famous as to warrant publication? I know of only one study. Peck (1988-1989) reported on a diary left by a 48-year-old woman who killed herself. He presented extracts from the last week of the diary to try to illustrate that her suicide was rational, that is, that she had the ability to reason, a realistic world view and adequate information, and that she was avoiding harm and achieving goals.

Peck was not convincing in arguing that these criteria are met, but the extracts from the diary he provided do mention the stressors that the woman was experiencing, her low self-esteem, her perception of herself as ineffectual and inadequate, and the pain, both physical and psychological, that she was experiencing as a result of her situation.[4]

1.4 Discussion

This chapter has reviewed examples of studying suicides in literature in order to generate and confirm clinical hypotheses about suicide, and of using the writings of suicidal authors to gain a deeper understanding of their motives for self-destruction. Although there are those who reject such uses for literature (e.g., Jaffe, 1967), a good test of these strategies is whether our understanding of suicide is increased, and I hope that the examples provided in this chapter have convinced the reader of their usefulness. I have also introduced studies of the suicide notes and diaries left by suicides and, in the following chapters, in order to throw light on the psychodynamics of suicidal behavior, I will examine in depth the diaries, letters, poems, suicide notes and other documents written by suicides.

4 A stroke had left her partially paralyzed, and a traffic accident had resulted in leg and facial injuries. She suffered from severe headaches after these events. She was also in love with a man with whom she was living who did not love her in return.

2 The Use of Computer Programs for Analyzing Suicide Texts

The vast majority of previous research on texts written by suicides has focused on suicide notes, and most of this research on the content of suicide notes has used judges to identify the presence or absence of content in the note. This requires subjective judgments which can be validated by looking at the inter-judge agreement between the two or more judges used. The advantage of this technique is that the researchers can decide what content categories are most relevant to their hypotheses, and they can have their judges score the content for these categories. In contrast, computer programs are typically devised to score texts for predetermined categories which may or not be pertinent to the researchers' hypotheses. Computer analyses tend, therefore, to be purely empirically-oriented rather than theoretically-oriented.

Several earlier studies have used computer programs to analyze suicide notes. Ogilvie, et al. (1965) compared a sample of genuine and simulated notes written by men and found that the genuine notes had more references to "things" such as roles and objects, whereas the simulated notes had more references to emotional states. Ogilvie, et al. also carried out more detailed analyses They examined sentences referring to the female role and found that the writers of genuine notes gave fewer instructions to females, gave more information about females, and made more references to being acted upon by females than the writers of simulated notes. Looking at the instructions given to females, the genuine note writers gave more specific instructions and fewer vague instructions. Looking at actions, the genuine note writers used the word "think" in the context of knowing or decision making (I think that if I went to the doctor, I would.....), whereas the simulated note writers used the concept more in the context of solving a problem (I am thinking of all the problems we have shared). Using three items (references to concrete things, places and persons; the use of the word love in the text; and the total number of references to processes of thought and decisions), Ogilvie, et al. were able to correctly classify 30 of the 33 pairs of genuine and simulated notes. Of course, this result needs to be replicated on a new set of genuine and simulated suicide notes to check on its reliability.

Henken (1976) also compared genuine and simulated suicide notes and notes written by people about to die using a computer program. The genuine notes were more concrete, constricted and concerned with interpersonal relationships (especially those with people of the opposite sex). Edelman and Renshaw (1982), using computer analysis, found that the genuine notes were longer and had fewer positive modifiers, more negative existential density (e.g., "not"), more negative authority (e.g., proper nouns), more negative audience (e.g., "you"), more modified nouns, more modified verbs, more negative generalized others (e.g., third-person pronouns), more cognizance of objects (concrete objects), more modification of objects and actions, more negative modification of unknown people, more static action, and fewer references to future time. To be honest, most of the differences identified seem to me to have little psychodynamic relevance.

The present set of studies uses a computer program (the LIWC; Pennebaker, et al., 2001) that, while still lacking a theoretical basis, does score texts for interesting content. The program has been used in a variety of studies of texts so that there is a body of research already published using the program. Many of the chapters in this book use the LIWC to study suicide notes, letters and blogs written by suicides, diaries from suicides, poems written by poets who died by suicide, and the words used in tapes recordings from suicides. The studies include both cross-sectional studies (such as comparing the suicide notes of men and women) and time-series studies (such as how the content of a diary changes over time.

2.1 The Linguistic Inquiry Word Count (LIWC)

The LIWC has been used to analyze many documents, including the narratives online by women with breast cancer (Bantum & Owen, 2009), the value of written essays about trauma in helping trauma victims cope (Klest & Freyd, 2007), the differences between truthful and deceptive language in prisoners (Bond & Lee, 2005), the differences between essays written by psychiatrically disturbed and normal individuals (Junghaenel, et al., 2008), personality differences in self-narratives (Hirsh & Peterson, 2009), and differences in the interviews between writers and physicists (Djikic & Oatley, 2006). There are also a large number of, as yet unpublished, doctoral dissertations that have used the LIWC. The LIWC has been adapted for use into Dutch (Zijlstra, et al., 2004), German (Wolf, et al., 2008), Korean (Lee, et al., 2006) and Spanish (Ramirez-Esparza, et al., 2007).

2.2 The Use of the LIWC for the Study of Suicide

Prior to this set of studies on texts from suicides, several studies have appeared using the LIWC. Pennebaker and Stone ((2004; see Chapter 3) studied the diary of a young women who completed suicide and found that the proportion of words indicating positive emotions increased as Katie came closer to the time of her suicide while the proportion of words indicating negative emotions decreased. Religious words increased while words related to death decreased.

Williams (2007) compared suicide notes from attempted and completed suicides and found no differences in words indicating belongingness and burdensomeness. In diaries, words indicating belongingness did not change over time, but words indicating optimism, certainty and causality increased as the suicide approached. Suicidal students did use more words indicating burdensomeness in their essays as compared to nonsuicidal students, but did not differ in words indicating belongingness. Also comparing suicide notes from attempted and completed suicides, Handelman and Lester (2007) found that the notes from completed suicides had fewer metaphysical references, more future tense verbs, more social references to others, and more positive emotions than did the notes from attempted suicides.

Stirman and Pennebaker (2001) compared the poems of nine poets who completed suicide with those of nine poets who did not do so. They differed in words indicating hopelessness and integration. Regarding hopelessness, it was predicted that the suicides would have more words indicating negative emotions and death and fewer words indicating positive emotions. Only the difference in death-related words was significant. Regarding integration, it was predicated that the suicides would have more self-references and fewer references to communication with others. The suicides did have more first-person singular words (e.g., me and my), but no differences in references to others, first-person plural words (e.g., we) or communications words. Over time, the suicides used first-person plural words less often. Although it was not predicted, the suicides did use more sex-related words throughout their poems than did the comparison poets.

Rogan (2009) studied the audio-transcriptions of words used in four crisis negotiation incidents. Two perpetrators surrendered to the police, while two completed suicide after releasing hostages. Several significant differences were identified. In the suicide incidents, there was fewer words related to anger, inhibition, seeing, and physical being. Predictions made on the basis of clinical knowledge about suicides (such as words indicating positive emotion, sadness and depression and personal pronouns) were not confirmed.

More recently, Stack, et al. (2012) compared suicide songs written by twenty four groups (such as Metallica and 3 Doors Down) with the neighboring track on the CD using the LIWC. The suicide songs were quite similar in content to the comparison songs except for two differences: the suicide songs had more words per sentence and a higher percentage of sad words, but they did not differ in other emotions or in references to death and suicide. Stack et al. concluded that the great degree of similarity explains why research exposing individuals to suicide songs has found no impact on their suicidal ideation, and why suicide songs *per se* do not appear to precipitate suicidal behavior. Any impact of the music of a group appears to result from the overall style and content of the group's music and not to any particular song.

Lester (2012) used the LIWC to compare the written memorials on online bereavement websites written by those who have lost a significant other to suicide and those who have lost a significant other from other causes. He found that the memorials written by suicide survivors were longer (and used longer words). They had more references to death, fewer references to themselves or to the deceased, and more words reflective of anger and sadness. He concluded that deaths from suicide have a more profound impact on the survivors and result in greater emotional distress than do natural deaths.

Many of the chapters, especially on those on the diaries left by those who died by suicide, use my subjective, qualitative interpretation. For the published diaries, readers can obtain a copy of the books and explore their own interpretation of the psychodynamics of the writer. For the personal diaries I have obtained from their significant others, only Katie's diary is available. The last month of this diary appears in Lester (2004b). I do not have permission to share the diaries of Jim (Chapter 6) or Robert (Chapter 7).

I use the LIWC in many of the following chapters, but I report only the significant trends and differences that I identified. The complete list of variables measured by the LIWC is shown in Table 2.1. Apart from the word count and the words per sentence, the other measures are expressed as percentages. For example, the measure for anger is the percentage of words expressing anger relative to the total word count. It is possible, of course, for a particular word to fit into two or more categories. For example, a swear word may also be a sexual word. The results of the LIWC analyses in each chapter are usually presented as Pearson correlation coefficients for ease of interpretation. Correlation coefficients can go from -1.0 to +1.0 and are often used as a measure of effect size.

Tab. 2.1: The LIWC categories, with examples of words.

word count
words per sentence
sentences ending with ?
unique words
words in the dictionary
words longer than six letters
abbreviations
emoticons
pronouns
First person singular (I, me)
First person plural (we, our)
total first person
total second person (you)
total third person (she, them)
negations (no, never)
assent (yes, ok)
articles (a, the)
prepositions (on, from)
numbers (one, thirty)
affective or emotional processes
positive emotions (happy, good)
positive feelings (joy, love)
optimism and energy (pride, win)
negative emotions (hate, worthless)
anxiety or fear (afraid, tense)
anger (hate, kill)

continued **Tab.2.1.:** The LIWC categories, with examples of words.

sadness or depression (cry, sad)
cognitive processes
causation (because, hence)
insight (think, know)
discrepancy (should, would)
inhibition (block, constrain)
tentative (maybe, perhaps)
certainty (always, never)
sensory and perceptual processes
seeing (saw, view)
hearing (heard, listen)
feeling (touch, hold)
social processes
communication (talk, share)
other references to people (pronouns)
friends (pal, buddy)
family (brother, father)
humans (boy, woman)
time (hour, day)
past tense verb
present tense verb
future tense verb
space (around, over)
up (above, over)
down (below, under)
inclusive (with, include)
exclusive (but, except)
motion (walk, move)
occupation (work, boss)
school (class, student)
job or work (boss, career)
achievement (goal, win)
leisure activity
home (house, kitchen)
sports (football, game)
television and movies (TV, sitcom)
music (song, CD)
money and financial issues (cash, taxes)
metaphysical issues (God, heaven)
religion (church, rabbi)
death and dying (dead, coffin)
physical states and functions
body states, symptoms (heart, cough)
sex and sexuality (penis, fuck)
eating, drinking, dieting (eat, swallow)
sleeping, dreaming (asleep, bed)
grooming (wash, clean)
swearing (fuck, damn)

Part I: **The Study of Diaries**

3 Katie's Diary[5]

Serendipitously, I was given a diary of a young woman who had killed herself. I have named her "Katie." The diary covered the last year of her life and was in five separate books. The diary was given to me by her younger sister, "Laura," who had never read the diary. Laura thought that, as a suicide expert, I might find it interesting. I was astonished. I had in my hands a source of data on suicide that was extraordinarily rare. Compared to a suicide note of a paragraph or two, I had over two hundred single-spaced pages of introspection! I had the opportunity to look into the mind of a suicide in greater depth than ever before, and perhaps it would be possible to obtain insights into the suicidal mind that conventional research has failed to provide.

I thought of colleagues who could read this diary and comment on it from their differing perspectives, and I explained to Laura that I could produce a book based on this diary, a book that would serve as a memorial to Katie and would contribute to our understanding of suicide. Laura permitted me to embark on this project, the result of which was *Katie's Diary: Unlocking the Mystery of a Suicide* (Lester, 2004a). The aim of the project was to explore what new insights into suicide an in-depth examination of the diary of a suicide could provide.

Ellis (2004) analyzed the diary from the point of view of a cognitive therapist. He was able to document dichotomous thinking, cognitive rigidity, hopelessness, deficient problem-solving, perfectionism, and dysfunctional attitudes in Katie's writings. Pennebaker and Stone (2004) used the LIWC program to analyze the diary, the same program that has been used throughout the present book. Pennbaker and Stone noted several trends over time in the diary. The five books were characterized, in order, as: (1) focusing on family history, with extreme sorrow and pain, (2) anger and self-abuse and a concern with her body, (3) feeling strong and in control, (4) anger at self, lack of control and disconnecting from people, and (5) loss and pain.

The number of entries declined over the year, but the length of the entries peaked in the first and fifth books. Many of the variables examine by Pennebaker and Stone did not show monotonic trends over the year, but rather peaked or had troughs at various points during the year. However, for the last six months, the proportion of words reflecting positive emotions increased, while the proportion dealing with negative emotions decreased. The use of question marks rose in the last six months, while concern with eating declined. Religious words increased over the whole year while death words declined for the first six months of the diary. Pennebaker and Stone, however, did not carry out statistical analyses of the trends they uncovered.

---

5 Part of this chapter is based on Lester (2004a).

3.1 Katie

Katie's parents had emigrated from Europe to the United States. Her father was German and her mother Hungarian. The father, a carpenter, was a domineering husband, preventing his wife from learning English and from driving a car, for example. He was an alcoholic and abusive to his wife and children. Katie was the first-born child, followed just over a year later by a sister, Laura.

Katie's father sexually abused her. In her diaries, Katie refers to this abuse, but does not give explicit details. It is possible that she does not remember the incidents clearly, but she may also be reluctant to describe the incidents in detail in her diaries. It seems reasonable to conclude that the sexual abuse involved genital and oral sexual acts. I do not know whether Laura, Katie's younger sister, was also sexually abused by her father.

Katie's mother threw her husband out of the house when Katie was nine years old. He sometimes returned to the house while the mother was out working (at a factory), and his daughters would have to call the police to have him removed. Two years later, when the mother was filing for a divorce, he died, possibly of a heart attack. Soon thereafter, the mother became schizophrenic. The state authorities decided that she was not competent to raise her two daughters who were then placed in foster homes. Katie's mother received inpatient care and was released but, after living in the community for eight years in squalid conditions[6], she was institutionalized in a state psychiatric hospital with her younger daughter named as her legal guardian.

The two daughters were placed in several foster homes during the next few years, only occasionally placed together. They went to different colleges in the state, Katie two years ahead of Laura. They kept in touch and were quite close. Laura felt that Katie was somewhat immature, and she became protective of Katie as the years passed.

Katie developed an eating disorder at the time that she was taken away from her mother and placed in foster homes. Her anorexia was severe enough that she was hospitalized on several occasions, often around the time of Christmas. She was also frequently depressed. There is no indication that Katie had attempted suicide in the past. The daughters had been raised as Catholics, but Katie developed eccentric religious ideas to the extent that Laura worried that Katie suffered from hallucinations.

Katie blamed her mother for the trauma that she had experienced, and she saw her mother as having been purposely vindictive to her children. She preferred to tell others that her mother was dead. Laura, on the other hand, loves her mother and does not hold her responsible for the trauma she suffered at the hands of her father.

From the diary, we learn that Katie has a boy-friend whom she loves, Mark. Their relationship is troubled. Mark seems to have had sexual intercourse with an

6 She failed to pay her real estate taxes and utility bills, so that she lived without heat and water, and she was unable to hold a job.

ex-girl-friend while he was seeing Katie, and this causes anguish for Katie and friction between her and Mark. Katie has trouble getting good grades in her college courses, and she sometimes withdraws from courses before the semester ends. She has financial problems paying for her college education and in getting a job to help with the finances. For the period covered by the diaries, Katie is overweight, and she is discouraged about this, continually trying to lose weight, but without success. She refers to attending group meetings for those who are overweight and for those who were victims of incest. She also mentions drinking and using recreational drugs, including marijuana.

On June 29, Katie's boyfriend Mark went to her college dormitory room (a single-story dormitory for disabled students[7]), but Katie did not respond. The light was on in the room, and Mark could see under the door that Katie was lying there. Mark went outside and broke the window so that he could enter the room, and he found that Katie had hung herself using a cloth belt hooked around the metal door-closing mechanism. Others in the dormitory called campus security who in turn called the local police department. There was no disorder in the room, except for the broken window, and there were no signs of foul play. No suicide note was found.

Mark reported that he had last seen Katie on June 16 and that she had recently been depressed. No one in the dormitory had seen Katie for the last few days. However, an employee of the bookstore had seen Katie on the day before her body was found. The autopsy report indicated that Katie was 20 years old and 65 inches tall and weighed 143 pounds.[8] There were no signs of any illness, disease or trauma apart from the hanging. Toxicological analyses revealed no alcohol or drugs. The medical examiner did not report examining Katie's reproductive system, and so it may be assumed that she was not pregnant.

3.2 The Ophelia Complex[9]

> ...When down her weedy trophies and herself
> Fell in the weeping brook. Her clothes spread wide,
> And mermaid-like awhile they bore her up,
> Which time she chanted snatches of old lauds,
> As one incapable of her own distress,
> Or like a creature native and indued
> Unto that element. But long it could not be
> Till that her garments, heavy with their drink,

7 Katie had moved to this dormitory after having disagreements with her roommate.

8 Katie's weight was within the range for a woman of her height with a large frame. It was outside the range for women with small or medium frames.

9 This discussion of Shakespeare's Ophelia owes a great deal to the written commentary provided to me by Kenneth Tompkins, my colleague at The Richard Stockton College of New Jersey.

> Pulled the poor wretch from her melodious lay
> To muddy death.[10]

In Shakespeare's *Hamlet*, Ophelia seems to have no mother. Hamlet woos the motherless girl, but her father warns her not to trust Hamlet at all. Obediently, Ophelia repels Hamlet's advances. As Hamlet's personal troubles develop, he admits to Ophelia that he loved her once but says that he no longer does. He gets angry at her and tells her to go join a nunnery. Later in the play, Hamlet inadvertently murders her father (who is hiding behind a curtain in the bedroom of Hamlet's mother). Ophelia goes mad[11] after the loss of her father. As she wanders around the castle and its grounds, it is her father's death that is on her mind. At one point, she climbs on a tree, and she falls into the river when a branch breaks. She makes no effort to save herself, but floats downstream until her wet clothes drag her under. In essence, she chooses suicide.

Tompkins noted that Ophelia is a "creature" designed by men. In her first appearance in the play, she is questioned by her brother, Laertes, about Hamlet's intention and urged not to have intimate relations with Hamlet. Later, after Laertes has left for Paris, Ophelia's father asks her about Hamlet's intentions and tells her to avoid Hamlet. Ophelia tells her father that she will obey. Her next appearance is merely to confirm Hamlet's apparent madness to her father. As Jardine (1983) observed, Ophelia is under the total control of both her father and the king, Claudius. For example, they order her to return Hamlet's gifts to her so that they may observe his reaction, and she obeys. She is used as bait so that they can observe Hamlet's emotions.

Hamlet is no better. He uses Ophelia merely to further his plans to expose his uncle as a murderer. If Hamlet really loves her, then she is chaste but, if he does not love her, than she is lewd and lascivious for accepting his gifts. Either way, she should go to a "nunnery" (which could mean a convent or a brothel). Jardine also noted that, if Hamlet married and had heirs, then they would inherit the throne. On the other hand, if Hamlet remained unmarried and without heirs, then Claudius and his offspring are the heirs to the throne. Thus, it is in Claudius's interests to have Hamlet break off his engagement to Ophelia. Female sexuality, therefore, represents "...woman's intolerable interference with inheritance..." (Jardine, 1983, p. 92). No one in the play cares about Ophelia–what she wants, what she feels or what she thinks.

McGee (1987) has pointed out that Ophelia is presented by Shakespeare in a way that would not endear her to Elizabethan audiences. There are clues that she is a Roman Catholic, and England then had its own "Church of England." Furthermore, the innuendo in the play is that Ophelia is also a whore. (Ophelia is described as mermaid-like as she drowns in the river, and mermaid was a slang term for prostitute.) Ophelia's madness is connected with the Devil, for she has displayed sexual feelings

10 The quotes are from Shakespeare (1969).

11 R. D. Laing (1960) considered her madness to be schizophrenia and so is evil. Had she lived in Elizabethan England, she might have been labeled a witch and subjected to an exorcism or killed. In one conversation with Ophelia, Hamlet says

> I have heard of your paintings too, well enough. God hath given you one face, and you make yourselves another. You jig, you amble, and you lisp; you nickname God's creatures and make your wantonness your ignorance. Go to. I'll no more on't; it hath made me mad.

Painting is a metaphor to suggest prostitution. Whores painted their faces to cover the ravages of smallpox and other venereal diseases that caused disfigurement.

Ophelia, then, has suffered the loss of her mother and has become an obedient daughter, but the loss of both her father and Hamlet's love leaves her ungrounded and unable to continue to live. (Had she not killed herself, she would also have experienced the loss of her brother in a short time too since he dies in the fight with Hamlet.) Furthermore, no one is concerned for her well-being, but rather they manipulate her to serve their own well-being.

It was not I, but rather Mary Pipher (1994) in her book *Reviving Ophelia* who suggested the relevance of Ophelia for understanding adolescent girls. Pipher presented cases of adolescent girls she had counseled who were depressed, suicidal and self-mutilating, anorexic and bulimic, abusing drugs and alcohol, sexually promiscuous and victims of sexual harassment and rape. Pipher argued that Ophelia chose suicide because she was not able to grow. She became the object of other people's lives and lost her sense of self, if she ever had it. Her development was thwarted, and her potential truncated.

Pipher noted that girls between the ages of seven and eleven rarely come to psychotherapy, not because these years are "latent" in the psychoanalytic sense, but rather because girls this age are interested in the world. They can be and do anything they want without worrying what others are thinking about them or how others are judging them. They can be their natural selves. But once adolescence arrives, along with puberty, the girls lose their resiliency and optimism. They are no longer curious, and they begin to avoid risks. Their assertiveness leaves them, their energy declines, and they become more deferential, self-critical and depressed. Pipher notes, too, that menstruation occurs at an earlier age today than it used to, and so the stress of adolescence begins at an earlier age. In addition, daughters stay at home longer, often until they finish college at the age of twenty-two, and so adolescence ends at a later age.

Ophelia in Shakespeare's *Hamlet* followed this path. After she fell in love with Hamlet, she became dependent upon his approval. Lacking inner direction, she tried to meet the demands of Hamlet and her father, Polonius, and the struggle to win the approval of both tore her apart. When Hamlet rejects her because she obeys her father, she drowns herself. Ophelia epitomizes the plight of adolescent girls today. Adolescent girls today encounter a world which demands that they subjugate their real selves and conform to the ways required of them in the society. But the life-style demanded of them is full of contradictions, contradictions so great that all cannot be met.

This split between the real self and the facade self, as I have called it (Lester, 1995b, 2010a), begins early in life when the parents demand that the child suppress particular desires and introject those of the parent instead. "Finish your food," "Be polite," "Do well in school," and all of the other demands made by the parents as they socialize their child create this split between the real self and the façade self. Almost all Western theorists of personality have described this phenomenon, although they use different terms to described it: introjected desires forming the superego in psychoanalytic theory, conditions of worth by Carl Rogers and the pattern of vicarious living by Andras Angyal, to name a few.

Pipher has pointed out that present-day culture now extends this. In the past, to be sure, parents continued to socialize their daughters well into adulthood, but girls typically had a large extended family nearby, sometimes living in the same house, which provided support and praise for them as they really were. They were, nonetheless, monitored closely and shaped to be "feminine" in the traditional sense of the word so that they would be found attractive by a young man and become fine wives and mothers. However, today, this continued socialization, with its accompanying suppression of the real selves of the girls, is taken over by the peer subculture and reinforced by the media. An extended family living nearby is rare, and the parents often both work and provide less support for their daughters.

This is made worse by the high frequency of divorce, which removes some of the parental influences and introduces even more chaos when the parents remarry and re-divorce. Drugs are much more freely available today than they were fifty years ago, adolescents engage in sexual intercourse at a much earlier age than in the past[12], and girls are encouraged by the media to focus on their bodies and their looks and to minimize their intellect. Pornography is everywhere, in videos and in song lyrics, and the media reinforces the thin, anorexic look, all the while running articles on the dangers of eating disorders.

If adolescent girls remain true to their selves, then their female peers ostracize them, and the boys ridicule them. On the other hand, if they conform to the sexy stereotype that the peer culture and media reinforces, then they run the risk of joining subcultures that use alcohol and drugs and encourage early sexual intercourse. In the course of this, they may be raped and then ostracized for being a "slut." Adolescent girls have to play dumb, be cute and pretty, and act sexy, yet resist the overtures of the boys who are "turned on" by this image.

Adolescent girls diet when they are hungry and when they should eat; they spend time with the "in-crowd" rather than with the friends they prefer; and they act dumb when they could excel academically. Interestingly, now parents tend to fight for their

---

12 Indeed, sexual intercourse was not an option for adolescents fifty years ago.

daughters real selves, but they lose out to the cultural and peer pressures. In addition, our culture remains sexist and misogynist. Pipher browsed through magazines in the 1990s available for young girls, and they all had articles on make-up, weight-loss, and fashion. Attracting boys was the sole goal in life, and the magazines had no articles on hobbies, careers, politics or academic pursuits. Pipher noted four ways of adapting to these pressures: conform, withdraw, become depressed, or get angry. Thus, the difficulties of adolescence, including extreme and changeable emotions and irrational thinking (which, of course, persists into adulthood, as cognitive therapists inform us), are made more difficult for adolescent girls.

All parents must love their daughters and give them affection. Pipher suggests that girls who make the best adjustment have parents who are not laissez-faire. Laissez-faire parents leave their daughters to make decisions that they are not capable of making wisely, and these girls often adjust worst. Parents who are very strict and controlling have daughters who traverse adolescence with the least trouble but who, as adults, have little sense of their real selves. A lot of affection and moderate control enable daughters to go through adolescence with some stress but with the chance to explore their selves and gain a sense of who they really are and what they really want. They function better when they are adults. "I love you, but I have high expectations for you" is the message parents should give. "We want you to explore and have fun, but we are setting limits too."

3.3 Katie as Ophelia

Katie had an alcoholic and abusive father. In her diary, she makes it clear that he molested her sexually, although she is not explicit about the details. (Perhaps she still has difficulty remembering the abuse?) It is likely that he raped her since, in one memory, he is described as replacing his clothes:

> June 8: People did such bad things to me when I had no clothes on.
> June 24: I felt so misused already, like a piece of meat, like I was when my parents did things to me.
> July 22: I remembered my father making me go on the bed naked with him
> July 24: ...hands he caressed with.....rubbing my rape away.
> July 19: ...his hands on my body again.....I saw him put his shirt on after he was done with me.
> August 28: ...pillow over my face–hands and mouth on my breasts.
> September 3: I think something happened in my father's car–I really don't know.
> January 1: ...I remembered something with hay, (bloody) old barn.....Daddy at the dresser, don't tell Mommy–me in bed, played with her lingerie. Maybe he dressed me up in it.

In such families, not only does the girl lose her father (since he wants her as a lover, not as a daughter), but she often also loses her mother. The mother may have (consciously or unconsciously) opted out of the sexual relationship with the father and promoted her daughter as a substitute sexual partner, or she may deny the sexual relationship between the daughter and the father. The daughter, therefore, can turn to no-one for help. She becomes, as it were, an orphan. Katie's mother had been physically and sexually abusive toward Katie also:

> June 14: I don't need my mother in my life anymore. I never needed someone who was so sick and raped me–my mind, my heart, soul.
> August 28: I'd beat her with the leather strap until she bleeds. The one she beat me with, and I'd kick her till she falls down and has the wind knocked out of her and kick her in the stomach like she did to me. I'd degrade her and make her take off her underwear and hold it into her face and tell her she was a whore and a slut and a bitch like she did to me.

Then, when the father left home (and died), Katie's mother become psychotic.[13] Katie and her sister Laura were placed with separate foster families.

Katie had several boy-friends, but her relationship with Mark was the most intense, and he was her first lover. The sexual molestation caused tremendous conflicts in her sexual relationship with Mark.

> June 8: I also have had such a problem with sex. I really don't like it that much. I really never want to do it.
> June 17: Mark and I made love this morning. It was nice.
> June 24: We made love. It was really beautiful.
> June 28: I like it when he gets rough with me.
> July 4: We made love for 2 hours. It was really nice.
> July 5: I can't have sex with him anymore. It is too much for me emotionally.

Then Mark is unfaithful to Katie by having sex with an ex-girl friend, Claudia, an act which further impairs Katie's trust in him.

> July 4: ...he told me he didn't love me as much as Claudia. Well, they were both sick and fucked in their relationship.

She can no longer be sure that Mark will remain faithful to her. Indeed, it is interesting to wonder whether Katie might have been better able to cope with life if she had not become involved with Mark. He stayed with her and professed his love for her during the year of the diary, but he was unfaithful early in their relationship, was jealous of her male friends, occasionally hit her, and behaved impulsively at times (for example, slashing his wrists). He broke up with her continually, although they always got back together. With her history of sexual abuse, Katie may not have been ready to handle sexual intimacy yet. But she also says:

---

13 She remains in a psychiatric hospital today.

> October 17: I don't know where my heart would be if I never met him. I honestly think I would've killed myself by now for some reason.

Katie's situation, then, is very similar to Ophelia's. She has lost both her father and mother, and she cannot be sure of Mark's faithfulness and love for her. And like Pipher's adolescent girls, Katie is depressed, has an eating disorder and mutilates herself.

> July 3: Weekend, drugs, alcohol, food binge.
> July 4: I abuse myself now–mutilate, destroy, manipulate, lie, control (sickens).
> July 5: I missed class today.....No more alcohol, pot, binges, lying.
> July 17: I want to slash up my whole fucking body right now.
> July 25: I wish I studied for algebra this weekend.
> July 28: I had to withdraw from college algebra again.
> August 17: Stealing sometimes is a must for me.
> September 11: I ran in front of a car so it would hit me.....I got up and said you're right and cut my wrist. Then he ran over to stop me and then he started screaming–saying he was sober–and started cutting himself. I fought him physically to make him stop and get the knife away. I tried every tactic I knew to make him stop. He cut himself, so the only way I made him stop was I started cutting myself. I cut my breast and my shoulder.
> November 1: I cut my wrist like a complete idiot. I stopped and thought, but did it anyway.
> November 22: I'm not going to eat all day.
> November 28: I talked, screamed and banged my head so hard yesterday.

3.4 Women, Depression and Rumination

In discussing Alfred Adler's theory of personality, Mosak and Maniacci (1999) noted that some individuals who develop psychological disturbance "cling" to their trauma. Many of us experience trauma during our lives, but we manage to recover from the shock and continue with a relatively normal life. Others do not. "They 'nurse it, rehearse it,' go over it again in their minds again and again, and ruminate about it, as if they were enslaved by the thought. By clinging to the shock effect, they create an excuse for not moving on with life" (Mosak & Maniacci, 1999, p. 123). The question becomes, therefore, why do some people cling while others let go?

One possibility has been suggested by Nolen-Hoeksema (1987) who suggested that women are, in general, more often depressed than are men because they have a ruminative response style which amplifies and prolongs their depressive symptoms. Rumination involves focusing on the symptoms of distress ("I am so tired") and on the meaning and the consequences of this distress ("What's wrong with my life?" and "Why me?"), trying to figure out why you are depressed, crying to relieve tension, and talking to friends about the depression. Rumination interferes with taking action and effective problem-solving, and individuals who ruminate tend to recall relatively more negative events from their lives which makes them more pessimistic about the future and helps perpetuate the depression. Individuals who get into this state also are more likely to lose social support because their behaviors alienate their friends, relatives and significant others. In contrast, Nolen-Hoeksema argued that men are more likely to get involved in distracting activities when they are depressed, activities such as going to movies or playing sports.

Nolen-Hoeksema thought that the ruminative response style in women is a result of the particular ways in which girls are socialized in the society and because women have lower status and power than men (Nolen-Hoeksema, Larson & Grayson, 1999). As a result of this lower status, women experience more negative events in their lives than do men, and they have less control over their lives, both at work and at home in their families. For example, even though some women work full-time, they are still expected to perform the majority of the child-care and domestic work in their families. This lack of control over their lives leads women to be more likely to develop a more generalized expectation that they are unable to control their lives and that they will never will able to do so. This makes the depression deeper and more chronic.

The role of rumination in depression is supported by research. For example, Nolen-Hoeksema and her colleagues (1987) studied a sample of residents in the San Francisco area and found that measures of chronic stressful events, depression, rumination and feelings of mastery over events were all inter-related and predicted depression a year later. Sakamoto (1998) in a sample of Japanese students found that self-preoccupation (the tendency to focus on the self), especially when measured for both its degree and duration, predicted the level of depression of the students.

The role of ruination is relevant here because sitting alone, writing a lengthy diary, probably increases the tendency to ruminate. Indeed, many times as I read Katie's diary, I wanted to tell her to stop writing and instead go out and socialize with other students at the university.

3.5 Resentment and Dependency in the Suicidal Individual

Many years ago, as part of my dissertation research, I administered the Situational Resources Repertory Test (RES Test) to suicidal and nonsuicidal individuals. The RES Test was devised by George Kelly (1955). The respondent is asked to think of 22 examples of specific crises in his or her life and then asked to which of 21 significant others he or she could have turned to for help. Kelly was interested in how people distribute their dependencies, and he thought that it was healthier if we spread our dependencies around more people. On the RES Test, this would mean that the person could call on more people for each crisis.

I wrote the names of the 21 significant others on cards and had the students sort them into seven piles of three each, from the three they liked most to the three they liked least. After completing a questionnaire, I then asked each student to sort the 21 significant others into seven piles of three each, from the three they resented most to the three they resented least.

The results were obvious to me before I carried out the statistical analysis. When I asked the nonsuicidal students to sort the significant others for resentment, most told me just to reverse the sorting they had done earlier for liking. (I made them sort by resentment anyway.) Hardly any of the suicidal students made this objection. They sorted by resentment without any quibbling, and the people they liked most were often the people they resented most!

When I did the statistical analysis, I confirmed this observation (Lester, 1969). The suicidal students resented those they liked and also those upon they depended. On the other hand, the nonsuicidal students did not resent those whom they liked, nor those upon they depended. Furthermore, the suicidal studentss had a smaller dispersion of dependencies, that is, there were fewer people to turn to for help in crises. The result was that the suicidal individuals more often were dependent upon a small group of people toward whom they felt much resentment. Thus, in times of crisis, it is likely that the suicidal individuals would be less able and less willing to turn to others for help because of these feelings of resentment.

Katie displays a great deal of resentment toward Mark and her friends. Her diary is full of ambivalence about the people in her life. About her boy-friend Mark, she states that she loves him and that she hates him, sometimes in entries for the same day. June 8th: I love Mark. June 15th: It's all a facade with Mark. June 24th:.....even though I've been angry at Mark and said I hated him, I never meant it.

The presence of conflicting feelings is also striking.

(1) June 14: I don't need my mother in my life anymore. June 17: I miss my Mom. June 24: You selfish cunt. I need a Mommy......I've never loved anyone except my Mom like this.
(2) Katie plans to spend time with a friend, Carl. But on June 22: I really almost hate Carl.....[Carl] is a total jerk actually.
(3) June 24: I can't wait to be alone in the house, doing my work. I love it. June 24: [later] I'm so alone.
(4) June 24: I feel very beautiful and strong right now. July 1: My body is against me.

In fact, it hard to find a person or an issue about which Katie does not express ambivalence. There are only two examples. Katie says only nice things about her sister, mostly about how much she misses her; and she says only harsh things about her father.

This ambivalence reminds me of George Kelly's theory of personal constructs. Personal constructs include those we use to evaluate other people. Is this person trustworthy or untrustworthy, intelligent or stupid, etc? Kelly postulated that constructs were bipolar, that is, each time we evaluate a person, she is either intelligent or stupid, never somewhere in between. Constructs are dichotomous judgments–either/or. I have always wondered whether this was in fact the case, but Katie's diary convinces me that, at least for Katie, her constructs were dichotomous and bipolar. Her judgments of people and experiences switches from one extreme to the other.

Shneidman and Farberow (1957a) proposed that suicidal individuals were prone to dichotomous thinking, and Charles Neuringer published a number of research studies which documented this (see Neuringer, 1988). He found that suicidal individuals more often thought dichotomously than did nonsuicidal individuals, and that they quickly switched judgments about people from one pole to the other. In particular, Neuringer and Lettieri (1982) showed that this was true for suicidal women, and Neuringer concluded that:

> It augurs poorly for the futures of these women. Dichotomous thinking imposes inflexibility and polarized thinking on suicidal individuals. It may be that the inflexibility and polarization associated with dichotomous thinking are what perpetuates and maintains for long periods of time a high level of crisis. If the above is true, highly suicidal women are caught in a web that appears to be seamless and never-ending.....If the cognitive style does indeed constantly keep the "emotional pot" boiling, it may explain why suicidal individuals feel so hopeless and why they have such difficulties envisioning a future in which they will feel better. (Neuringer, 1988, p. 51).

3.6 Positive Disintegration

Many years ago, Dabrowski (1964) introduced the notion of *positive disintegration.*

> In relating disintegration to the field of disorder and mental disease, the author feels that the functional mental disorders are in many cases positive phenomena. This, is, they contribute to personality, to social, and, very often, to biological development. The present prevalent view that all mental disturbance are pathological is based on too exclusive a concern of many psychiatrists with psychopathological phenomena and an automatic transfer of this to all patients with whom they have contact. (p. 13)

Dabrowksi noted that the recovery of some patients results, not only in the recovery of their health, but also the attainment of a higher level of mental functioning. There is here, then, the recognition that some crises and some disintegrations of the personality can have a positive growth effect. The person may be unable to grow, perhaps, if disintegration is prevented.

Gut (1989) has touched on the same theme in her book *Productive and Unproductive Depression*. She argues that depression can serve an adaptive purpose for the individual. The withdrawal and lowered mood which accompanies depression allows the person to dwell on their conscious and unconscious processes and perhaps resolve deadlocks in their functioning.

What makes depression unproductive rather than productive? Gut suggested that a person who has been overtaxed in the past will be more likely to have unproductive depressions. This can be caused by early trauma and by family functioning that prevented understanding and resolving these trauma. There may be no one to whom the individual can communicate the depression and despair and with whom the feelings and accompanying thoughts can be discussed. There may also be genetic predispositions and social and cultural factors that make productive resolution of depression difficult.

It is clear that the early trauma experienced by Katie, particularly the sexual abuse by her father, which was then followed by the schizophrenic breakdown of her mother, were the kinds of experiences which would have made a productive resolution of her depressions difficult, if not impossible.

Gut felt that finding a good listener was critical in resolving depressions productively. While writing a diary helps some depressed people (or writing letters, praying or meditating), a live listener is much better. It is interesting that, despite the large number of people referred to by Katie in her diary, none of them appear to be good friends, that is, the kind of person with whom one can sit down and talk exhaustively about a problem of concern. Katie's only confidante is her boy-friend Mark, and she is too dependent upon (and conflicted about) that relationship for Mark to be the ideal confidante. (We might note also that we have no evidence to evaluate whether Mark himself is capable of being a good confidante for someone who is depressed or in distress.)

3.7 Discussion

Many years ago, Binswanger (1958) treated a woman, Ellen West. At the time that he treated Ellen, psychiatrists did not understand the disorder that we now refer to as anorexia, an eating disorder. Ellen was diagnosed as schizophrenic at the time, but the misdiagnosis did not matter that much since there were so few treatments available, if any. Psychotherapy was primitive, and medications unavailable. Eventually, Ellen killed herself. Binswanger, an existentialist wrote:

> .....I exist authentically when I decisively resolve the situation in acting.....In contrast to the "affect"-laden short circuit reactions of her earlier suicide attempts, this suicide was premeditated, resolved upon mature consideration. In this resolve, Ellen West did not "grow beyond herself," but rather, only in her decision for death did she find herself and choose. (Binswanger, 1958, p. 299).

> .....the existence in the case of Ellen West had become ripe for its death in other words, that the death, this death, was the necessary fulfillment of life-meaning of this existence. (p. 295)

> .....only in her decision for death did she find herself and choose herself. The festival of death was the festival of the birth of her existence. (p. 298)

Thus, Binswanger concluded that suicide was the correct and necessary path for Ellen West to take. I must confess that, as I read Katie's diary, I sometimes had a similar reaction.

But, like Carl Rogers (1961), I have also criticized Binswanger for his handling of the case (Lester, 1971a), accusing him of psychic homicide (Meerloo, 1962), that is, killing a difficult and incurable patient by propelling her to kill herself or putting her in a situation where the likelihood of suicide was great. Binswanger treated Ellen West as an object, and he failed to respond to her in a genuine and empathic way. Katie needed an intervention. By herself, despite her strengths, she was unable to change her life-path. She reached out to others, both friends and a lover. She went to groups for incest survivors and for those with eating disorders. She went to college and planned a career, perhaps in nursing (helping others). She wrote her diary. But all of this was not enough.

Katie needed a psychotherapist to guide her through this period in her life. But for many distressed individuals, a psychotherapist is not possible for reasons of accessibility and of cost. Had Katie found a therapist, perhaps at the college counseling center, if her college had such a center, she may not have "connected" with her psychotherapist or perhaps been restricted to brief short-term counseling which might have been insufficient. It is, however, regrettable that Katie was unable, for whatever reason, to find a psychotherapist to help her discover an alternative life-path, one which did not lead to suicide.

3.8 The LIWC Analysis

For the present study, the diary entries were first divided by the thirteen months over which they spanned, and correlations were calculated over the months (numbered 1 to 13). For the second analysis, the eight entries in the final book which covered the period from May 30th to June 20th (the final entry in the diary) were analyzed by day (numbered 1 to 8). Katie died on June 29th. The scores from the LIWC program were then correlated over the 13 months for the first analysis and over the eight days for the second analysis. The results are shown in Table 3-1.

Over the 13 months prior to her suicide, five significant trends were noted as well as nine non-significant tendencies. The entries were longer at the beginning of the year, but the wording was more stereotyped (there were fewer unique words). Katie was less interested in the causes of her distress as the year advanced and referred less often to the past. Finally, death words became less common toward the end of her life. Looking at the non-significant trends, Katie referred to others less often over the course of the diary, expressed less anger, focused more on eating (Katie had an eating disorder and she felt overweight for most of this year), and less on sexual matters. (Katie had been sexually abused by her alcoholic father and had difficulties in her sexual relationship with her boyfriend.) The content of the diary sounds more positive toward the end, and this is reflected by a tendency for positive emotions to be more common and negative emotions less common, so that the ratio of positive to positive-plus-negative emotions increased slightly (the correlation coefficient was 0.30).

Tab. 3.1: Changes in Katie's diary over time

	By month over the year (n = 13)	By day over the last month (n=8)
	Pearson r	Pearson r
Word count	-0.89**	-0.29
Unique words	0.63*	0.25
Pronouns	-0.51#	-0.58
Second person	-0.55#	-0.38
Negations	-0.48#	-0.02
Prepositions	0.53#	-0.09
Numbers	0.48#	0.31
Anger	-0.55#	-0.37
Causation	-0.56*	-0.19
Past tense verbs	-0.57*	-0.51
Music	-0.48#	-0.36
Death	-0.57*	-0.35
Sexual	-0.50#	-0.73*
Eating	0.50#	0.50

** two-tailed p < .001, * two-tailed p < .05, # trend (two-tailed p < .10)

These trends were, on the whole, present also in the last month of Katie's life. However, the small number of entries (only eight) resulted in few of the trends being significant. Death words became even less frequent in the last month, as did concern with sexual matters. References to the past became less common, and the emotions expressed continued to become more positive.

3.9 Final Thoughts

Katie's diary ended nine days before she killed herself, and she left no suicide note. In the light of these trends, which seem to indicate a more positive outlook on life, one wonders whether some traumatic event occurred in those final ten days that increased her suicidal intent, but we will never know. However, it is striking that her mood improved over the weeks and months, and this suggests that we should be careful in thinking that our depressed and suicidal friends and loved ones are doing better if their mood improves.

The trend toward the presence of fewer death-related words in the later entries of the diary fits with the hypothesis of Spiegel and Neuringer (1963) that people would tend to suppress thoughts of death and suicide as they came closer to the time of the action. They found this in a study of suicide notes, and there was a long-term trend in Katie's diary in this aspect.

In the later entries, Katie was less concerned with causation (perhaps less concerned with explaining her choices) and less concerned with the past. There was also less anger and less concern with sexual matters. Considering this, along with the increase in positive emotions and the decrease in negative emotions, we can hope that Katie found some measure of peace toward the end of her troubled life.

4 Cesare Pavese[14]

Diaries written by suicides are rare. However, occasionally a diary written by a famous person who has died by suicide is published, and the present study explored the final year of a diary written by the Italian novelist Cesare Pavese. Pavese's diary has been published in an English translation, thereby introducing two confounding elements, the translation itself and the fact that we cannot be sure that the editor of the diary did not omit some of the content. The Italian version is *Il mestiere de vivere* (Pavese, 1952), and an edited translation has appeared (Pavese, 1961). Cesare Pavese was born in Italy in 1908, and he killed himself at the age of 42 on August 27, 1950, in Turin, Italy. During that time, he became a leading intellectual, editor, translator, poet and novelist. The biographical details of Pavese's life are taken from his biographer, Lajolo (1983).

4.1 Pavese's Life

Pavese was born on a farm in Santo Stefano Belbo in the Piedmont province of North Western Italy (which borders on Switzerland and France) on September 9, 1908. He often returned to his hometown in later years. Pinolo Saglione, a carpenter there, remained a friend and confidante. Pavese's father Eugenio worked in Turin at the Court of Justice. Pavese's mother, Consolina, was the daughter of wealthy merchants. Consolina had lost three children before Maria and Pavese, the first dying of diphtheria at the age of six. Pavese had a sister, Maria, six years his elder. Pavese's childhood was spent in Turin during the Winter and Spring, and at the farm in Summer and Autumn. When Pavese was six, his father died from a brain tumor from which he had suffered since before Pavese's birth, and Pavese felt a great sense of loss, Lester (1989b) reported a higher incidence of loss of parents in the latency years (six to fourteen) of suicides, suggesting that early loss can sensitize individuals to later loss.

Pavese's mother, long tried by tragedy, was not warm or tender but rather showed her love by working hard for the family. She was thrifty and kept a tight rein on her children. She forbade talk over meals and forced the children to eat everything she served. Pavese began to withdraw from her, and their relationship became increasingly cold. He developed a lifestyle of being alone and detached, even when among others, and of feeling sad. At high school, his eyesight was poor, and he needed to wear glasses. He was tall, slender and frail, and walked with a slouch. He often had a bad cough in the winter, and he developed asthma.

Pavese rejected the political philosophy of fascism and, as fascism grew in popularity in Italy, he withdrew more into himself and his studies. At college, Pavese

14 Part of this chapter is based on Lester (2006, 2009).

seemed happier than ever before. He began to appreciate films and to translate American authors into Italian. His thesis was on Walt Whitman, and initially it was rejected because his professor viewed it as a political attack on fascism. Pavese managed to change advisors and graduate. Whereas Pavese's friends and colleagues were involved in the resistance against fascism and the political struggles after the Second World War, he rarely participated. He did not join the resistance during the war, as he stayed in the countryside, away from the fighting. He joined the communist party after the war but was never active.

Lajolo (1983), Pavese's biographer, noted that the people in Pavese's novels are vagabonds, drunks, and idle. The characters spend their lives in taverns, drinking and talking. They have no occupation, are without love, addicted to drinking and smoking, content to wander the streets aimlessly all night, and in the end they sink into melancholy. This was very similar to Pavese.

It is perhaps not true to say that Pavese did nothing. He wrote poems, novels and essays that intellectually supported left-wing ideas. Even his translations of American literature in the 1930s can be seen as challenges to the fascist regime by introducing Italians to the American ideals of freedom of thought and speech, and he worked tirelessly in these endeavors. He was exiled in 1935 for ten months by the fascists and was under surveillance for much of the time. But even Pavese knew that he was avoiding the real fight. At the end of the war, when he learned that friends had died fighting for the ideals he supposedly supported, his feelings of being a failure were amplified.

A few months after receiving his degree, Pavese's mother died. Although they had not been close, she had represented his roots and given him a sense of security. To replace her, he moved in with his sister and her family, where he lived sporadically for the rest of his life.

In order to earn some money, he translated American and English novels (1928-1932), wrote poetry (1932-1937), and eventually wrote short stories and novels. His first serous depression was after his exile in 1935 when he was crushed upon his return to Turin to find out that the woman he loved had just married someone else. His first book of poems had not been received with any enthusiasm, and he no longer saw writing as worthwhile.

He was drafted into the army in March 1943, having been previously excused because he was the son of a widow. However, when they discovered his asthma, he was sent to a hospital for six months convalescence. The fall of the fascist regime saved him from service. When he returned to Turin, most of his friends had left to join the partisans in the Resistance War against the Germans. Pavese went to stay with his sister in the country where he once more immersed himself in literature. His diaries from this period contain no mention of political events or the war. After the war, he returned to Turin and worked as before at Einaudi's, a publishing company. He found that many of his friends had died in the fighting. He finally joined the Communist Party, perhaps as a way of redeeming himself. He continued his writing but, after completing each book, Pavese would become physically weak, asthmatic, bitter and depressed.

In the late r1940s, Pavese was often nervous and anxious. He could not tolerate solitude in the city, so he hurried off to Santo Stefano Belbo, his old home, to visit with Pinolo Scaglione. His sister became accustomed to him disappearing every weekend. Suicide had been a constant theme in his writing and, in his novel, *Among Women Only*, published in 1949, he described the way in which he would later kill himself. He began to worry about headaches and whether he had a brain tumor like his father. He smoked medicinal cigars to ease his asthma. He wrote in his diary about his agitation, palpitations, a sense of decay, and insomnia. In June 1950, he was awarded the Stega Prize for his new novel, *The Beautiful Summer*, but he killed himself in August that year.

4.2 Women

After the poor relationship he developed with his mother, it is not surprising that Pavese had problems with women in his life, problems which became the major sources of his depression. Let us look at his first school-time crush, Olga. He tried to speak to her but felt too shy and inhibited. So he watched her from afar. He felt inferior to her, a simple country boy with big hands and poor vision, while his friends socialized with ease with their girl friends. One day he was walking by the river and saw a boat with the name Olga written on it. He turned white and fainted.

A second revealing incident happened while he was at the lyceum. One day, Pavese found the courage to ask a singer at a cabaret out. They set a date for six in the evening, meeting at the front of the club. Pavese arrived punctually at six. He waited and waited. At eleven, the rain began, but still he waited. At midnight he retuned home, sad, humiliated, and freezing. He learned the next day that she had left via the back door with another admirer. The depression and fever led to pleurisy, which lasted three months.

Later he would write much about his philosophy of life, in his letters, his diary, and his novels. He once wrote to a friend that no joy surpassed the joy of suffering. “That there can be a sort of pleasure in self-humiliation, is a fact” (May 9, 1936). We can see this clearly in his stubborn wait outside the nightclub for six hours. Lajolo is rather coy about Pavese’s love life. Perhaps he visited prostitutes. It certainly seems as if Pavese was impotent, most likely ejaculating prematurely and so rarely satisfying his lovers. It may also be, according to Lajolo, that his penis was small.

There were three major loves in his life, all of whom rejected him. Lajolo described the first love as “the woman with the hoarse voice.” She was studying mathematics at the university and was firm, cool, strong-willed, and good at sports. While he was with her, Pavese was more natural, human, tender and confidant than ever before. But she betrayed him, leaving him bitter and never again trusting woman. Lajolo does not tell us whether Pavese and this friend were lovers. Lajolo tells us, without giving examples, that Pavese rejected maternal or submissive women, as well as those that loved him. Rather he fell in love with and pursued those who did not love him, strong women with a mind of their own, perverse and unfaithful.

When Pavese was in exile, the woman with the hoarse voice rarely wrote to him. On the day he returned from exile, his friend Sturani met him at the train station. Pavese asked him about her. Sturani told him that she had been married the previous day. Pavese fainted. Although she married another, it is important to note that before Pavese's exile, her lover was in prison and they communicated by letters sent via Pavese. It was one of these letters for which he was tried and exiled. She had never been faithful to him, and Pavese had been willing to accept this! From the train station he went to his room in his sister's house and stayed there for days. He refused to eat, he did not read, and he thought of suicide. But he lived on.

In 1940, Pavese met Fernanda Pivano and was in love with her for five years. They met almost daily, and he would read her poems and novels. He asked her to marry him one day, but she did not reply. In all of those five years, Pavese never kissed Fernanda! Eventually she married someone else.

In Rome in 1945, Pavese met another woman who aroused his passion. Lajolo is again coy, and we learn nothing save that Pavese made an attempt to prove his virility. Dissatisfied, he returned to his silence and to self-destructive thoughts. Back in Turin he wrote, "You know you are alone? That you are nothing, and that is why she left you" (December 7, 1945).

The final woman in his life was an American actress visiting Italy, Constance Dowling. As soon as he met her, he began to fear her desertion. He realized that she was a flirt (and she did go to bed with a fellow actor). In July 1950 he was with her in Milan and appeared "blissful." Constance went back to America, and Pavese waited for a telephone call from her saying she would marry him. It never came.

Shneidman (1982) viewed Pavese as a manic lover, emotionally intense and obsessive, whose style frightened women away. This is incorrect. Pavese was an observer, a non-actor. He never spoke to his first love, Olga. He never kissed Fernanda in five years. Constance Dowling went back to America, and Pavese waited for her to call him. As for the "woman with a hoarse voice." Pavese passed letters from her to her lover and back. Indeed, in commentating on his fiction, Pavese wrote, "My stories are tales by an onlooker who watches things greater than himself take place" (February 21, 1942). His protagonists were replicas of himself.

One problem was that Pavese was attracted to flirtatious, untrustworthy women. "The only women worth the trouble of marrying were those a man cannot trust enough to marry" (September 27 ,1937). You must not let your "loved ones know the pleasure it gives us to be with them, otherwise they leave us" (September 30, 1937). "Women are an enemy race, like the Germans" (September 9, 1946). It seems that he was attracted to women (affectionate but untrustworthy) who were the opposite of his mother (cold but trustworthy).

4.3 Depression and Suicide

Pavese became depressed early in his life. His failures with women exacerbated these feelings and precipitated the most severe depressions. Depression would also develop after he had completed a novel. Throughout his life he talked about feeling worthless, and he focused particularly on his failures with women. No matter how much he wrote or how enthusiastically his writing was received, he would compare himself with those who were married and had children and consider himself a failure. And his impotence! He wrote, "...a man who ejaculates too soon had better never been born. It is a failing that makes suicide worthwhile" (September 27, 1937).

He described his life as a fight with depression, one that he had to fight "every day, every hour, against inertia, dejection, and fear." In 1927, he wrote to his friend Mario Sturani saying that he was incompetent, timid, lazy, weak and half mad. Should he kill himself or not? But he didn't have the courage to kill himself. He said that was a child, a cretin, a 'poseur.' More probably, he said, he would masturbate himself to death. Don't cheer me up, he wrote. Let me enjoy my depression in peace.

While he was at the lyceum, a friend, Baraldi, and his girl friend went to the mountains where they shot themselves. Baraldi died; his girl friend lived. Within a few days, Pavese decided to imitate Baraldi. He took a gun to the same town, Bardonecchia, but could not kill himself. He fired the shots into a tree instead. Pavese does not seem to have attempted suicide again prior to his death.

Pavese thought of suicide as a comfort in times of pain, but he thought of himself as a coward because he did not act on the thoughts and kill himself. "My basic principle is suicide, never committed, never to be committed, but the thought of it caresses my sensibility" versus later "...a futile dolt, proposing himself up with thoughts of suicide, but not committing it" (April 10, 1936).

In August 1950, his sister, staying in the country, was worried about her brother, so she returned to Turin. She found him frighteningly thin, his eyes hollow and red. For two days he burned letters, documents and photographs. He left his light on all night, but then became calm, patient and even kind. On the morning of Saturday August 26th, he asked Maria to pack him a suitcase as if he was going away for one of his weekend trips. He went to the hotel Roma in town. On Sunday evening, a hotel employee was worried because the guest had not been seen all day. He forced the door open and found Pavese lying on the bed dead, dressed except for his shoes. On the nightstand were sixteen empty packets of sleeping pills. His last words in his diary read, "All this is sickening. Not words. An act. I shall write no more" (August 18, 1950).

Shneidman (1982), in his analysis of Pavese, noted his use of oxymorons in his diary, the juxtaposition of opposites. "We obtain things when we no longer want them" (October 15, 1940). "The richness of life lies in memories we have forgotten" (February 13, 1944). Such stylistic writing does not necessarily portend suicide. Pavese's diary is not a daily record of events, but rather a set of pensees and, as a writer, Pavese no doubt devised and treasured these clever thoughts.

In discussing death and suicide, Shneidman noted that Pavese seemed to confuse the self as experienced by the self with the self as experienced by others. "Then it is conceivable to kill oneself so as to count for something in one's own life?" (January 16, 1938). Yet it is likely that Pavese's suicide did add stature to his reputation and that he does, even now, count for more than he would have had he died from natural causes.

Today, Shneidman would focus more on the psychological pain that Pavese suffered—the psychache (Shneidman, 1996). "Loneliness is pain; copulation is pain; piling up possessions or herding with a crowd is pain; Death puts an end to it all" (January 19, 1938). Shneidman also noted that much of Pavese's writings seem to reflect constriction of thought and dichotomous thinking. Success and failure were extremes to be contrasted, as were having a woman love you and being totally alone.

4.4 Discussion

Pavese's disposition and childhood experiences (the death of his father and his unaffectionate mother) prevented him from becoming mature. He never left home, moving from mother to sister, living most of his forty-two years with them. He never developed the social skills necessary for relating to women. He behaved much like an adolescent in first encounters with girls.

Pavese had friends, but listen to what he says, "As soon as I am aware that a friend is getting too close, I abandon him. I abandon women, those whom you call maternal, as soon I deceive myself into thinking they love me." Pavese cannot stand closeness. It scares him. At another time he writes, "Pavese wants to be alone–and he is alone–yet, at the same time, he yearns to be in the center of a group which is conscious of his solitude." He is alone, even when with friends. Indeed, his intellectual concerns about literature, which formed the topics for his conversations and his many essays, are ideal ways for having intellectual contact with others while remaining emotionally distant.

His fears over his impotence were probably unfounded. It is possible that the little sexual contact he had made premature ejaculation more likely. With more sexual experience (and less anxiety over his sexual performance), his sexual behavior might have become more normal. But the initial failures led to shame and to anxiety that he would always fail, and the shame and anxiety probably made him fail in the future. It became a self-fulfilling prophecy, a prophecy made more likely by falling in love with women who rejected him. It is hard to make love to a woman who hurts you and toward whom you feel anger.

Pavese suffered from depression all of his life. He frequently thought of suicide and eventually killed himself. It is a wonder that he lived so long and was as creative and productive as he was. Lajolo gives us no hints of a history of depression in Pavese's family. Though Pavese lost his father when he was six, his father had been ill all along, and so the death may not have been unexpected. His mother was cold, but she clearly cared for her family. Pavese's childhood was not ideal, but was far from being as traumatic as some childhoods.

What Lajolo and Shneidman have missed is the connection between rejection by woman and Pavese's denigration of his literary work. From the start of his diary, Pavese showed no confidence in his work. "The day came when my vital stock had been entirely used up in my works and I seemed to be spending my time merely in retouching or polishing" (undated, 1935). "In other words, there is a blind spot in my work as a poet" (October 9, 1935). "I have fallen short of resigning myself to total failure" (March 29, 1946). "I have fallen short of the standard I should have reached" (November 9, 1935). But what is interesting is how failure with women leads to such thoughts. On April 10, 1936, in the same short paragraph, he wrote, "Even my period as a woman-hater (1930-1934) was in essence self-indulgent I have never really worked and in fact I have no skill in any occupation." In a later paragraph that day, he wrote:

> I have had a love affair during which I have been judged and pronounced unworthy to continue. In the face of this cataclysm, I feel not only the pangs of a lover, agonizing though they are; not only the break-up of our association, serious as it is; but in my mind the whole thing becomes confused with a sensation of being hammered by life, a feeling I have not known since 1934. Away with aesthetics and poses! Away with genius! Away with the low! Have I even in my life done anything that was not the action of crack-brained fool? (p. 48-49)

On March 26, 1938, Pavese wrote:

> What use has this long love affair been? It has uncovered all my short-comings, tested my quality; passed judgment on me. Nothing is salvaged. Conscience is shattered: look at my letters and homicidal temptations. My character is warped; look at my imprisonment. The illusion of my genius has vanished; look at my stupid book and my translator mentality. Even the hardihood of the ordinary man in the street is lacking. At thirty, I cannot earn a living. (p. 100)

This sequence of thought was made easy because "My stories are always about love or loneliness" (August 30, 1938). As years passed, the pattern continued. Pavese began 1946 with enthusiasm. "You have power, you have genius and something to do" (January 1, 1946). But an affair ended: "She has always followed her caprices and her own conveniences... and now she is gone" (March 1, 1946), whereupon "...all I have to say is already said...[I] cannot resign myself to total failure" (March 29, 1946). Again, toward the end of his life, Pavese writes of his latest book on November 17, 1949, "It is certainly my greatest exploit so far...You also have the gift of fertility...You are as famous as any man can be who does not seek to be so." Yet as he gets involved with Constance Dowling, he writes, "I am filled with distaste for what I have done, for all my works" (January 14, 1950). After she leaves him, to fly back to America, on August 17, 1950, in the penultimate entry in his diary, Pavese wrote, "In my life I am more hopeless, more lost than then. What have I accomplished? Nothing." Once a woman rejects him, then his writing loses all value. It would be interesting to know how his mother responded to her son's literary aims and early poems.

Using Judith Beck's (1995) formulation of a cognitive perspective for disturbed behavior, the triggering events (in Pavese's case, rejection by a woman) activate his core belief that he is basically incompetent as a writer. The acclaim with which his work is greeted (even the literary prizes he was awarded) was not able to overcome his core belief. In Aaron Beck's (1991) theory, these core beliefs are called core schemas, systems of related beliefs that give us consistent ways of perceiving and responding to situations, schemas which can be triggered by external or intrapsychic events.

Kovacs and Beck (1978) described how the separate thoughts in a person's mind become linked so that one thought almost always leads to the next thought. They illustrated this with the case of Mr D. While interacting with his wife, the thought came to him, "I am unable to respond to my wife emotionally," followed by "I'm alienated from my family," and "I'm responsible for my wife's depression." Another sequence was identified in which approval of others gave Mr D a sense of worth, and he needed the approval of others to justify his existence every day. If this approval was not received, then he thought that he was not entitled to approve of himself and so he did not have the right to exist. A therapist, who has accurate and detailed knowledge of a client can diagram this sequence. Kovacs and Beck called these thought complexes *schemata*. Pavese's diary provides examples of such cognitive schemata.

Binswanger (1958), in discussing the case of Ellen West, an anorexic who eventually died by suicide, argued from an existential perspective that only in her death did she become an authentic person, acting rather than being acted upon by other forces. Pavese thought, "The worst thing a suicidal type of man can do is not killing himself, but thinking of it and not doing it." On November 6, 1937 he finally killed himself. The observer, the person who never behaved decisively, finally did so.

4.5 A Text Analysis of Pavese's Diary

The last year of the Pavese's diary, from August 18 1949 to August 18 1950, was divided into thirteen segments by month, and the 13 segments were scored by the LIWC program. Fifteen significant associations were identified at the 5% level of statistical significance or better, which is more than would be expected on the basis of chance (see Table 4-1).

As the diary entries approached the month of Pavese's suicide, the sentences had fewer words, the proportion of words found in dictionaries increased, the proportion of long words decreased, the use of first-person singular pronouns increased as did references to the self, there were fewer articles (such as "the") and prepositions, there were more positive emotions and optimism, more tentative words (such as "perhaps"), more future tense verbs, there were fewer including words (such as "with"), and fewer references to occupations, schools and jobs.

Most interestingly, the analysis replicated the finding in Katie's diary that positive emotions became more common as the diary entries get closer in time to the suicide (see Chapter 3 above). However, in the case of Pavese's diary, negative emotions did not decline as they did in Katie's diary. Furthermore, in Pavese's diary, there was no change in religion-related words, but there was a trend toward an increase in death-related words.

The increase in positive emotions over Pavese's year is noteworthy in two respects. First, not only does it replicate the finding in Katie's diary, but it parallels changes found in an analysis of a series of letters written by a young man who killed himself to a friend over a period of two years (see Chapter 11 below) where negative emotions were less often expressed in the letters as the time of the young man's death approached. Katie's diary had changes in both positive and negative emotions, Pavese's diary a change in positive emotions, and the young man's letters a change in negative emotions. This suggests that a useful measure in future research might be the ratio of positive to negative emotions.

Tab. 4.1: Correlations documenting changes in the content of Pavese's diary over the last 13 months of his life (numbered 1-13)

	Pearson correlations
Words per sentence	-0.58*
Words in the dictionary	0.57*
Words longer than 6 letters	-0.70**
Emoticons	-0.61*
First person singular	0.72**
Total first person	0.71**
Articles	-0.66*
Prepositions	-0.55#
Positive emotions	0.55#
Optimism	0.61*
Tentative	0.64*
Future tense verbs	0.64*
Inclusive	-0.67*
Occupations	-0.63*
School	-0.56*
Job	-0.63*
Metaphysical	0.52#
Death	0.51#

two-tailed p < .10, * two-tailed p < .05, ** two-tailed p < .01

Second, as I noted in Chapter 3 above, the changes in emotions prior to an act of completed suicide has been noted in the twenty-four hours prior to the suicide from clinical notes on psychiatric inpatients who killed themselves while in the hospital (Clements, Bonacci, Yerevanian, Privitera & Kiehne, 1985; Keith-Spiegel & Spiegel, 1967). This suggests that these changes may occur to some extent over a longer period of time.

The other changes in Pavese's diary suggest the unique individual character of changes. Diary entries may change in some ways that are common to many suicides, as well as in ways that are unique to the individual's own life circumstances. In Pavese's case, the diary entries became less complex (shorter sentences and fewer long words) and more self-oriented.

The many changes identified in this study confirm that meaningful changes in the content of the diaries of suicides may be observed in translation and possibly even in edited diaries.

5 Arthur Inman[15]

Arthur Inman was born on May 11th 1895 in Atlanta, Georgia, the only child of rich and prominent residents. He died by shooting himself on December 5th 1963 in his home in Boston. He left a diary of approximately 17 million words, some of which has been typed and microfilmed. An abbreviated version of the diary was edited by Daniel Aaron and published (Aaron, 1985), amounting to 1599 printed pages in two volumes. Aaron accomplished an incredibly difficult task and is to be commended for his effort.

Unfortunately from the point of view of a suicidologist, Aaron was a Professor of English and American Literature and Language, and he chose what to include in the published volumes on the basis of throwing light on the social and political events of the time, albeit from one person's perspective. In particular, the edited extracts end in 1951 on page 1526, and the last 12 years of the diary are omitted except for very brief extracts of no more than a few pages. The missing years are probably of little interest to a social historian, but crucial to a psychologist trying to understand the reasons for Inman's suicide. This chapter is a qualitative analysis of the parts of the diary that have been published.

There have been four brief commentaries on Inman, and most of the commentators disliked the man. Aaron (1985) called him a "repulsive weakling," Shneidman (1994) talked of his repellent attitudes and warped personality, while Maltsberger (Leenaars & Maltsberger, 1994) described him as selfishly indulgent and corrupt. I disagree. If any of us kept as detailed and honest a diary as Inman did (17 million words in some 50 years), recording *every one* of our thoughts, desires, emotions and dreams, none of us would appear to be "nice" individuals. Inman's attitudes and desires can be found in most people, but others do not record them for us to read. For example, of course Inman was a racist and a sexist, but so were most people born in the South in the 1890s (as well as in the 20th and 21st Centuries all across America). Had he stayed in Atlanta and become a successful businessman, he might well have joined other similar men and co-founded the Augusta National Golf Club! Indeed his political views (such as liking Joseph McCarthy and disliking Franklin Roosevelt) can be found today in commentators such as Ann Coulter.

In this chapter, I will first briefly described Inman's life and then try to understand the reasons for his suicide, except that I think that the interesting question is not why did he kill himself, but rather why did he *not* kill himself much earlier in life. I am often impressed by how long suicides live rather than puzzled by their deaths. For this essay, I have based my analysis on the two-volume published edition of the diary (Aaron, 1985) and commentaries by Leenaars and Maltsberger (1994) and by Shneidman (1994).

---

15 This chapter is based on Lester (2010b).

5.1 Inman's Life

Inman went to local schools until he was 13 whereupon his parents sent him to board at the Haverford School outside of Philadelphia where he was bullied and spent five miserable years. The bullying seems to be have been traumatic for Inman, although he did not have a breakdown until his college years. It has been well-documented that bullying can have a serious impact on mental health (Srabstein, 2008) including suicidality (Kim 2008).

His parents then sent him to Haverford College, although he would have preferred to begin a career back in Atlanta. Despite enjoying college life to some extent, he had a physical and nervous breakdown in his third year and dropped out. There may have been some experiences at college which re-aroused the trauma of the earlier bullying at school, but Inman does not mention any in his diary which he began a few years later. He stayed in Boston for the rest of his life, convinced that he was very sick and treated by a team of osteopaths who realigned his bones and organs, pumped his stomach, administered enemas and prescribed several dangerous chemicals for him (especially bromides). His father supported him financially, although not excessively but upon, his father's death in 1951, Arthur inherited substantial assets. From 1920 on, he lived permanently in an apartment in Garrison Hall in the Back Bay area of Boston where he paid a succession of staff to assist him as he lived out his life in darkened rooms, sound-proofed as best he could. They cooked for him, massaged him, read to him and told him about their lives. Some let him cuddle them, caress them and have sexual intercourse with them. He met Evelyn Yates, a student at Wellesley College, and married her in 1923. They remained married (with occasional separations) until his suicide in 1963.

5.2 Inman's Illnesses

Musto (1985) read Inman's diary and provided a medical opinion on his health. The idea of auto-intoxication, that bacteria in the intestines were responsible for many illnesses, was a popular view in that era. Elie Mechnikoff, who was awarded the Nobel Prize for medicine in 1908, believed it, and it was an accepted medical theory. The osteopathic theory that misalignment of bones was responsible for many ailments was, however, not accepted by the medical establishment at that time.

Musto saw Inman's breakdown in 1916 as brought on by some minor medical problems which "allowed him to achieve some deep wishes to be alone but cared for" (p. 1609). Indeed, a year before his breakdown, Inman wrote that this was what he desired. Musto thought that Inman may have had "loose joints" but saw no reason why this would have caused pain and disability. Musto saw most of Inman's physical ailments as the result of his excessive ingestion of bromides and barbiturates prescribed by his "doctors" and his somewhat excessive use of alcohol. Bromide intoxication results in blurred vision, disordered sleep, and headaches, all of which Inman complained. Musto concluded that Inman did suffer from migraine headaches, hemorrhoids and nasal allergies, but the rest of his ailments could be attributed to his substance abuse and the medical maltreatment (especially the enemas with corrosive chemicals, stomach pumpings, and the ultraviolet radiation of his throat which resulted in sores).

5.3 Psychiatric Diagnosis

Maltsberger (Leenaars & Maltsberger, 1994) diagnosed Inman's breakdown at college in 1916 as a major depressive disorder with symptoms of crying fits, loss of energy, difficulty sleeping, loss of appetite and low self-respect. The result was a regression with Oedipal overtones–a close attachment to his mother with the father excluded. A psychiatrist whom Inman consulted in 1918 suggested that Inman be separated from his mother and placed in a sanitarium. According to Maltsberger, Inman encouraged his wife to socialize with his osteopath, "Dr. Pike" (with whom, unbeknownst to Inman at the time, she had an affair), and then tried to break up their relationship, thereby recreating and, this time, successfully resolving his Oedipal conflict (albeit unconsciously) by getting his wife back. Maltsberger, therefore, speculated that a significant trauma (which remains unknown to us) occurred for Inman between the ages of 3 and 6.

Leenaars (Leenaars & Maltsberger, 1994) focused on Inman's childhood as documented in the diary: a difficult birth, a domineering but loving mother, a father who wanted a girl, verbal and physical abuse from his father, and a horrible experience for five years at a boarding school far from home (from the ages of 13 to 18). Inman hated his father but loved his mother. On the other hand, there were no major traumata experienced by Inman in his early years until he was sent off to boarding school.

Maltsberger thought that Inman's mother was neurasthenic and that Inman identified with her. Indeed, Inman himself noted that she kept a diary and liked to advise and counsel others, just as he did (pp. 1569-1570). His depression appears to have persisted, resulting in suicidal behavior in 1941 and 1963. Maltsberger also diagnosed a narcissistic personality disorder. Maltsberger noted that Inman behaved as a small child, expecting the prerogatives accorded children. He was incapable of sustaining friendships but paid an array of servants and people to keep him company and run his errands. He was not only exploitive and selfish but also a psychological voyeur. He paid young women to come to his darkened bedroom where he probed their minds and caressed their bodies.

Maltsberger found no signs of psychosis in Inman, except for possible delusional ideas about his body, ideas which were promulgated by his osteopaths. Maltsberger felt that Inman's suicide was carried out in a state of acute visual hallucinosis that verged on delirium tremens caused by acute alcohol-barbiturate withdrawal possibly complicated by bromide poisoning.

5.4 An Analysis of Arthur Inman

5.4.1 Social and Political Views

Inman disliked Jews and African-Americans and wrote many derogatory passages about them. He also disliked the English, Irish and Slavs and even blue-eyed people! Yet one of his closest friends was an African-American woman, and his friendship with her changed his views considerably. Indeed what is remarkable in his diary is that Inman was able to admit occasionally the irrationality of his views and was able to find good qualities in some of those groups he disliked. There are also groups whom he admired, such as the Chinese and the Japanese.

He had strong political views (a style Aaron called a "paranoid style" of political thinking) and ended up disliking (even hating) most of the Presidents during his life. He admired "strong" leaders, even writing admiringly of Hitler, but he also admired Ghandi. However, he was quite clear that he would have hated to live as a German under Hitler. He was strongly anti-Communist, supported Joseph McCarthy's effort to root out Communists from the American government, and saw Stalin as a great danger to the world. These views were not atypical at the time, or even now, and do not indicate psychopathology. Most people, though, would speak carefully if they held such views and not write openly and emotionally about them in a diary that they intended to be published.

5.4.2 Arthur Inman's Goals in Life

Having settled into his cocoon-like existence, Inman had two goals. The first was to become a published and acclaimed poet. However, although he had a few poems published in newspaper and magazines, his books of poetry were published at his own expense (mainly in the 1920s) and never received critical acclaim.[16] He also edited the lettesr of George E. Pickett, a Confederate General in the American Civil War.

His second goal was to write the diary which he wanted to be published after his death. He wrote in it almost daily, then he edited each volume years later, and had much of it typed and then microfilmed. He set out to be completely honest in the diary – to record his life and thoughts uncensored. Even when he later regretted writing particular entries, he never changed them, even when he wrote about his wife or staff,

16 His efforts to write songs and plays were even less successful.

people who would read the entries later as part of their work. This makes the diary similar to one by someone who never intends to have the diary made public. Inman hoped that the diary would make him famous after his death, but many times he had doubts about the value of the diary and whether it would bring him fame. Periods when he thought it was brilliant were often followed by periods of self-revulsion.

He wrote about social and political events, content which he thought would interest later readers. He also paid ordinary people to come and talk to him about their lives (initially for $1 an hour) so that his diary is a record of the lives of people living in the 1900s. Despite his prejudices, people of all ethnicities and religions are included. In addition, several of his staff became particularly close to him, and he detailed their lives in more detail. It is this task that leads Maltsberger to label Inman a "psychological voyeur."

For many of his intimates, not only did he listen to them and record their lives, he tried to change them. He lectured them on attitudes and style. They turned to him for advice. He bought them clothes, changed their make-up, improved their speech and manners, and helped them set and achieve goals. The ends toward which he aimed were not always perhaps appropriate for his "pupils," and he was especially abusive (both verbally and physically) to his wife whom he hit in the early days of their marriage (acts which he later regretted and for which he apologized to her) and whose personality he could never accept. She was supposed to change to be the kind of woman he wanted, and he could not accept her as she was. A few of his intimates abandoned him after a few years and refused to ever visit him again, but others appreciated him and loved him, remaining close to him even after they married and moved away.

At the end of his life, a young 16-year-old girl ("Kathy Connor") moved into an apartment in his building. Aaron describes Kathy as pretty, poor, uneducated and Irish. Inman did cuddle and caress Kathy, but he never had sexual intercourse with her. Inman referred to Kathy as his "bewitching daughter." He loved her, and she loved her surrogate father. (Her parents had divorced when she was two and neglected her.) He turned her into a "lady," and when she went to work as a saleswoman at Newbury Clothiers, Inman would have her driven to work in his car and enter by the front entrance rather than by the staff entrance. Aaron says: "Today Kathy feels indebted to him for his efforts to make her think well of herself" (p. 1583). Several of his intimates felt this way about Inman. Maltsberger (1994) called him "unloved." This is not so. Even his wife, who had many fights with him, who separated from him from one brief period and who had a long-term affair with Dr. Pike that Inman knew nothing about at the time, loved him and was with him until his death.

In his interest in the minds and lives of other people and in his desire to change them for the better, I think that in modern times, with appropriate training, he might have made a good psychotherapist. After all, are not psychotherapists psychological voyeurs who wish to improve people for the better? Inman merely lacked the training and the appropriate setting for his goals.

Inman had many doubts about his goals. He was forced eventually to accept that he was not a good poet. He read published diaries of others so that he could compare his with theirs. This would sometimes convince him of the worth of his own diary, but he also worried from time to time that his achievement as a diarist were poor. Although Aaron did publish some of the diary, it is not apparent whether any scholars have used it since its publication. It is ironic that it is Inman's suicide that made the diary of interest for the present paper.

5.4.3 Sexuality

Inman's first sexual intercourse was in 1922 with a woman he had hired to read books to him. The first time had little impact on him, but he reported that his "devils danced a bit" (p. 211) the second time, whatever that means. He was not able to "relieve" himself, and the same happened the first few times he had sex with his future wife, Evelyn, also in 1922.

Inman and Evelyn married in November, 1923. Inman had a limited sexual life with his wife. At times, his diary implies that sexual intercourse became rare and, in the best of times, Inman wanted intercourse no more than once a week. After Dr. Pike died in 1949, and Evelyn told him (in 1950) of her long-term affair with him, their sex life improved for a while, but it soon returned to its limited state.[17]

Leaving aside the cuddling and caressing with young women, Inman did have a few affairs (the first in 1932). Inman's wife knew about these, and later even volunteered to buy contraceptives for the women. After 1951, when Aaron's systematic excerpts from the diary cease, Inman did have sex with "Lillian" who was 17 when Inman met her, and with whom he had an exciting erotic relationship. They continued to be lovers after Lillian got married until she and her husband moved to Arizona. Lillian was followed by "Martha" whom he met in 1949 when she was 17 and who stayed his lover until 1956. Thereafter, Inman contented himself with girls between the ages of 12 and 15 with whom he did not have sex but merely touched and was touched.

Maltsberger, as we noted above, zeroed in on the Oedipal conflict in Inman. Let us explore this in more detail. Inman does note that his father never masturbated, and Inman never mentions masturbation himself. He seems to have problems in sexual intercourse. He mentions never experiencing passion. The one time he had sex with one of the women who slept naked in his bed with him, he appears to have been unable to ejaculate. There is no mention in the diary of the quality or quantity of

17 In an entry in 1933, he wrote, "Curse my impotence" (p 519), but it is not clear whether this is a sexual reference.

sexual intercourse with his wife for him, but his wife found it unsatisfactory.[18] The majority of his interactions with the women was like those of a child – touching, caressing, fondling – he of them and they of him. He never mentions any occasions on which they masturbated him.

Maltsberger noted that Inman was close to his mother and saw his father as an enemy.[19] It is possible that Inman was a latent homosexual. One wonders whether the frail, slight, young Inman, sent off to the horrendous boarding school, was sexually abused by those boys who bullied him and what sexual role in life Inman might have chosen had he remained at home and attended local schools with peers who shared his social and subcultural background.

5.4.4 Stressful Life Events

Aside from his chronic pain and invalidism, Inman experienced a number of stressors during his life. Staff to whom he grew close (he often spoke sincerely of loving them) left. His poetry was consistently rejected for publication and judged to be poor. His mother died in 1933 and his father in 1951. His wife had breast cancer and a mastectomy in 1947.[20] After Dr. Pike's death in 1949, Inman learned of his wife's affair, and she left him in 1951, although she agreed to return after a few months apart. It is interesting than none of these events led him to plan or attempt suicide.

5.4.5 Finding a Meaning in Life

Victor Frankl (1963) proposed that the striving for meaning for one's life is a primary motivational force in people. The desire for such a meaning is as basic as the desire for power or for pleasure. Once we find the meaning, then life becomes more bearable. Following Nietzsche, Frankl noted that those who have a "why" to live can bear any "how."

Frankl noted that life has no general meaning. There is no abstract meaning that is true for all people. The meaning of life differs for each person and from day to day. Life has only a specific meaning for you at this moment. Each of us must find our own specific mission and concrete assignments in life. Each of us is questioned by life, and each of us must answer for our own life.

---

18 After the death of Dr. Pike, and his wife's confession of the affair, she coached him on how he should make love to her. However, she soon refused sex again, encouraging him to find satisfaction with other women, even though she admitted to mild jealousy (e.g., p. 1451)

19 He saw the male body as beautiful and the female body as "a weak collection of curves" (p. 273).

20 After this, she became more independent and stood up to Inman more than she had in the past.

How do we discover the meaning of our lives? Frankl suggested that we may do a deed of some kind and thereby achieve or accomplish something (creative values). We may experience a value, such as a work of nature or a cultural object or a person, as when we fall in love with someone (experiential values). We may suffer, and suffering is a very common path toward finding a meaning for life. We can face our fate without flinching (attitudinal values).

If life is meaningful, then all the parts of life have a meaning, including suffering. What is critical is the attitude we take toward suffering–the attitude in which we take our suffering upon ourselves. (This suffering must be necessary and unavoidable. A person who suffers from an illness because he refuses to get a cure from a doctor is suffering unnecessarily.) We can accept our fate (and our suffering) with dignity and with an unselfish attitude, or we can whine and rage. It is important to have right action and right conduct. Life ultimately means taking upon ourselves the responsibility to find the right answers to its problems and to fulfill the tasks that life sets us. We end up, therefore, not in a tensionless state, but with a striving and struggling for some goal worthy of us.

Inman found meaning in his work. He tried two paths – as a poet and as a diary writer. He failed as a poet, but he maintained a hope throughout his life that his diary would be found valuable after his death. Although he had doubts from time to time about the value of his diary, he always returned to his hope that it was indeed a worthy endeavor.

Inman suffered, both physical pain and psychache (Shneidman, 1996), and he communicated this to his wife, servants and companions. His diary perhaps served as an outlet, a place where he could write about his pain and, thereby, spare those around him some of his complaining. Frankl noted that it is the attitude that we take toward our suffering that can make the suffering meaningful, but it seems that Inman never found meaning in his suffering, and his suicide was an escape from suffering that appeared to Inman to have no meaning.

5.4.6 Suicidality

As Shneidman (1994) noted, Inman was chronically suicidal all of his life, with 50 or so entries on death and suicide from 1912 to his suicide in 1963. Inman was in great psychological pain throughout his life. Inman wrote about hating life in 1925, and wondered why he did not kill himself in 1927. He thought seriously about shooting himself in 1929 (his wife had hid his gun) and acquired chloroform and wrote suicide notes in 1934 (but decided not to kill himself). His depression was constant, and he often wrote that his life had been a failure (e.g., p. 941) and that he was a "nobody" (e.g., p. 914). Although he was good at manipulating people, he knew that it was his money that kept others close to him. He wrote that he lacked the fortitude to kill himself (e.g., p. 791)

In writing about his suicidal desires, he sometimes mentioned his aversion to noise in these early years and the pain from his medical problems. He wrote that, if his doctor (Dr. Pike) was no longer available, he would kill himself. He also laid the blame for his miserable psychological state on the five years he spent boarding at the high school. He often thought of himself as a failure.

> May 23 [1930]. I certainly am miserable, dispirited, downcast. My nerves are piling up for another migraine. I see double and that with pain. I wish to God I were dead. Once upon a foolish time I considered myself gifted with brains, endowed with some especial talent, given to thinking unusual ideas. Now I realize sadly that I am not unusually talented in any way, in fact a failure among failures, a nobody. (p. 415)

Inman's first suicide attempt was in 1941. Nothing much had changed in his life at that point except that the traffic patterns had changed on Huntington Avenue outside the apartment building in which he lived.[21] The noise and the traffic lights upset him and disturbed his sleep. On November 19th, he had his chief aide nail rugs over the windows, and he began to write of killing himself. (Remember that he lived most of the time in his darkened apartment, listening to books for the blind or having books read to him. His life was similar in some ways to living in a small dungeon.) On November 27th, he took an overdose of sleeping pills (nembutol and Veronal), and his aide found him at 7.30 am the next day. Initially, his wife left him without medical help until after 1 pm, and she argued with the doctors in the hospital to let him die. Inman declared himself proud of her. She never called him selfish, nor did she cry in front of him. Inman wrote on December 3rd, "I wish the doctors had let me die" (p. 1047). However, he did not attempt suicide again until 1963. He was pleased that he had the courage to attempt suicide, but he wished that the doctors had let him die.

In 1963, Inman's life continued in pretty much the same style, except that he was getting older and there was a major change in his living conditions. The apartment building in which he lived was very close to what became the Prudential Center. Buildings all around his apartment were torn down, and construction commenced on the 52-story building. The other change was that Inman's wife was drinking more heavily (she eventually joined AA), and Inman's consumption of alcohol also increased.

He took an overdose of sleeping pills in March 1963, was found by his housekeeper and ended up in Massachusetts General Hospital. Rather than move back to his apartment, he moved to an apartment hotel in Brookline. He could not adjust to the change, especially the new noises. Aaron described him as bored, irritable, nothing could distract him for long: not sex or reading or cuddling little girls. "I feel a harried ninety years old," he wrote, "with gathering pressures closing in about. I have lived too long. I have written too much."…..He confessed himself a failure and doubted that his work would survive – it would have been better for himself and everyone

21 There was some ongoing stress in his marriage, but this was present throughout their marriage.

connected with him if he had died in 1941....On December 4 [1963] he reported: "This has truly been a session in hell. Eight migraines yesterday, and one more at six this morning, with violent headaches and nausea." (p. 1598)

Inman knew that overdoses would not bring certain death, and so he shot himself on December 6th 1963.

5.5 Discussion

Arthur Inman lived 68 years. For all of his adult life, he was in chronic intense physical pain, and he lived a severely restricted life – staying in his darkened apartment almost all of the time. He had an unsatisfactory marriage, and those he paid to attend to him and to whom he grew close left him after a few years of service. He aspired to be a successful poet, but failed. He hoped that his diary would bring him fame after his death, but he often doubted that it would. The only pleasures in his life seemed to come from the books that were read to him[22] and political news, and from his interactions, social and sexual, with others. He experienced several stressors (parental deaths, marital rifts, and the loss of close friends), but he weathered these well.

What precipitated his suicide attempt in 1941 and his death in 1963 was the disruption to his life caused by the noise and chaos near his apartment. The tremendous change brought about by the construction of the Prudential Center was the stressor that he could not survive. He could not face leaving his "cocoon" in order to live elsewhere. One wonders whether, had the Prudential Center not been built, how long he would have lived. I suspect that he would have died from natural causes.

Stack and Wasserman (2007) applied Agnew's (1992) General Strain Theory to suicide. Agnew described several economic-related strains, including economic goal blockage, economic loss, and economic noxious stimuli. The category of economic loss included loss of property including one's home. Of the 675 suicides studied, Stack and Wasserman found evidence of economic-related strains in 67 suicides, and ten of these suicides had loss of a home as a precipitant. Inman's home was a tremendously important, secure and safe place for him, and the prospect of losing it was catastrophic for him.

What is surprising is that this "repulsive weakling," "warped personality" and "corrupt" individual should have lived so long and that the noise of construction and traffic should have precipitated his suicide. Indeed, it is impressive that he was able to construct a life that was full and during which he helped, with both advice and financial support, so many other people.

Pennebaker (1997) has shown that writing about emotional and traumatic experiences has a beneficial impact on physiological functioning (such as immune function),

22 He also listened to recorded books.

behaviors (such as work performance), and mental health (see also Lepore & Smyth, 2002). Pennebaker speculated that writing has these impacts because of self-disclosure and because of cognitive changes such as reduced rumination and increased assimilation of unexplained experiences. Most diaries are written privately, and only the writer reads them (at least while the writer is alive). Inman's diary differs in this respect. Not only did his wife read the entries, but also Inman employed members of his inner circle to type his handwritten diary (and eventually to microfilm it). Thus, those about whom he was writing often read what he wrote about himself and about them. Inman's diary, therefore, had the importance component of self-disclosure which is considered to be a beneficial therapeutic tactic (Jourard, 1971).

Lester and Terry (1992, 1993-1994) suggested, in discussing the lives of poets such as Anne Sexton and Sylvia Plath, that their poetry may have enabled them to continue living. Had they not been able to express their inner most thoughts and emotions in their writing, they might have killed themselves much earlier in their lives. It is possible, therefore, that it was Inman's diary that enabled him to live. In addition to giving his life a purpose (providing a record of his times that he hoped would bring him posthumous fame), it also gave him an outlet for his thoughts and emotions, a way of ventilating and exorcizing his inner demons and, in this way, enabled him to continue living.

6 Jim's Diary[23]

Jim died on September 6, 2004, at the age of 36. He was raised in a small, farm town and was the youngest of four children. His father was a truck driver, and the family lived frugally. Jim used marijuana and had only passing grades in high school. He joined the army where he met his future wife. She left him after a few months of marriage and Jim attempted suicide by overdosing on aspirin. His treatment at that time focused on his poor relationships with a distant and cold mother and a passive and uninvolved father.

After discharge, he lived in an apartment close to home, took courses in information sciences but never graduated. He worked the night shift in a hospital computer department. His father died when Jim was 30, and he spent the next year assisting his mother. He met a woman from Malaysia over the Internet, lived in Malaysia for 18 months with her, and then they both moved to the States where Jim got a job with computers. The woman eventually moved back to Malaysia because of a break-up over Jim's drinking. Jim bought a house, but lost his job after of a company merger. He took a substantial severance package and did not look for work. Jim eventually became short of money, and his car registration and car insurance expired.

Jim's sister tried to help him address his losses and get counseling for his alcohol abuse. He did stop drinking for a week, but then relapsed. She arranged a family intervention for him, but Jim refused to attend. He began to hide from his family, and his family members had little contact with Jim except for a few brief e-mails. Jim expected that he would soon have his utilities cut off and lose his house. He decided to kill himself, and he used a method that can be found on the Hemlock Society website – a plastic garbage bag and a rubber band. He died in his house, and a worried neighbor alerted the police who investigated and discovered him on October 2, 2004, 26 days after his death.

Jim began his diary on January 24, 2004 and entitled it "Drinking Diary." The original intent was to log the time of his drinks so that he would have a record of his alcohol intake. He also documented his food preparation and eating habits. An additional area of heavy commentary involved his activities with computer games, music, television and movies. He spent most of his time at home, sleeping during the day and awake at night. He spent a great deal of time recording and watching television and movies, listening to music, playing computer games, and surfing the internet. He maintained a website that provided pictures and reviews of local rock bands playing in nearby bars. Attending these "gigs" and e-mailing friends and family were the bulk of Jim's social life. As time progressed, his entries became more reflective about his life and his wish to end it.

---

23 This chapter was co-authored by David Lester and Cheryl Kaus.

Tab. 6.1: The number of words in each segment of the diary

	Words	Words per day
January-February	9914	275
March	15708	506
April	16352	545
May	22677	732
June	30977	1033
July	34489	1113
August-September	48778	1318

This chapter explores the psychodynamics of Jim's suicide through an analysis of his diary, and looks for changes as the time of his death grows closer. Two types of analysis were used: (1) a qualitative analysis by a psychologist, and (2) the LIWC computer program. The length of the diary is shown in Table 6-1.

6.1 The Qualitative Analysis

The journal was read by one of the authors for any content demonstrating Jim's reflections and concerns. Emergent themes were identified, and the entries were coded over the nine months. The entries for each theme were converted to percentages to reflect prominence within each month. Six themes had either high frequencies or interesting trends over time. These themes and their prominence per month are indicated in Table 6-2.

Tab. 6.2: Prominent themes over nine months (from the qualitative analysis)

Month	1	2	3	4	5	6	7	8	9
Suicidal thoughts	11%	7%	3%	23%	45%	39%	42%	47%	43%
Seeking connection with others	14%	32%	35%	11%	2%	14%	12%	0	15%
Seeking distance from others	0	0	11%	9%	6%	3%	6%	6%	1%
Helplessness, hopelessness, and worthlessness	32%	9%	0	17%	23%	21%	15%	12%	14%
Writing for an audience	0	.8%	0	0	4%	4%	6%	18%	14%
Stress and depression	11%	9%	5%	20%	2%	1%	6%	6%	2%

To display change over time in a more holistic way, the themes per month with at least 20% prominence are combined and presented below.

Month 1: Helplessness, hopelessness, and worthlessness (32%)

Month 2: Seeking connection with others (32%); attempts to stop drinking and make positive life changes (22%)[24]

Month 3: Seeking connection with others (35%)

Month 4: Suicidal thoughts (23%); stress and depression (20%)

Month 5: Suicidal thoughts (45%); helplessness, hopelessness, and worthlessness (23%)

Month 6: Suicidal thoughts (39%); helplessness, hopelessness, and worthlessness (21%)

Month 7: Suicidal thoughts (42%)

Month 8: Suicidal thoughts (47%)

Month 9: Suicidal thoughts (43%)

In the last nine weeks of Jim's life, there were specific emphases that appeared:

(1) Extreme vacillation over to live or to die, together with a rationale:

(i) Reasons for living – Considering what he will miss, and what he won't experience in the future.

(ii) Reasons for dying – Insistence that he is not able to turn his life around.

(2) Insistence that alcohol was the escape from the reality that he cannot change and not the reason for ending his life.

(3) Loss of money, and therefore the loss of ability to buy alcohol and pay bills.

(4) Making preparations prior to suicide such as throwing things away and designating what to bequeath.

(5) Acknowledging that he was writing for an audience.

The specific emphases over the last nine days were:

(1) Plans to die in a week or two.

(2) Much vacillation.

(3) Hope for help and intervention up until 44 minutes before his final decision

(4) Self-condemnation.

(5) Specific messages to readers:

(i) Thank you.

(ii) Don't blame yourselves.

(iii) Requests and instructions

---

24 Attempts to stop drinking and make positive life changes was a theme that appeared only in Month 2 as a result of abstinence from alcohol for one week.

6.2 The Computer Analysis

The results of the LIWC analysis are shown in Table 6-3. The noteworthy findings are:

6.2.1 Changes over Nine 25-day Periods (numbered 1-9)

- Word count increased
- More references to self over time
- More references to "You" and to friends
- More positive emotions
- More anger
- Less anxiety
- More future-orientation and less past-orientation
- More focus on metaphysical issues and death
- Less preoccupation with body, eating and sleep
- More "discrepancies" (could, would, should)
- More tentative words (maybe, perhaps)
- More words of certainty (always, never)

6.2.2 Changes over the Last Nine Weeks (numbered 1-9)

- An increase in positive emotions
- An increase in optimism
- An increase in anger
- A decrease in anxiety
- Less past-orientation
- More concern with sports (the football season began)
- More concern with music
- More concern with metaphysical issues and death
- More swear words

6.2.3 Changes over the Last Nine Days (numbered 1-9)

- More mention of Jim himself and "you"
- More negations (no, never, not)
- More concern with cognitive processes
- More certainty
- Less past-orientation
- More present-orientation

Tab. 6.3: The statistically significant changes over time in the LIWC analysis

	Nine 25-day periods (1-9)	**Final 9 weeks (1-9)**	**Final 9 days (1-9)**
Word count	0.95	-	0.88
Unique words	-0.95	-0.68	-0.90
Words in the dictionary	0.68	-	0.67
Words longer than six letters	-	-	0.80
Abbreviations	0.77	-	-
Emoticons	-0.69	-	0.77
Pronouns	0.71	-	0.75
First person singular	0.75	-	0.79
Total first person	0.74	-	0.79
Total second person	0.83	-	0.82
Negations	-	-	0.88
Articles	0.79	-	-
Numbers	-0.78	-	-
Affect	-	0.75	-
Positive emotions	0.71	-	-
Optimism	-	0.73	-
Anxiety	-0.79	-	-
Anger	0.71	0.82	-
Cognitive processes	-	-	0.78
Discrepancies	0.73	-	-
Tentative	0.84	-	-
Certainty	0.77	-	0.76
Senses	-0.88	-	-
Humans	0.91	-	-
Past tense verbs	-0.79	-0.74	-
Present tense verbs	-	-	0.67
Future tense verbs	0.74	-	-
Inclusive	0.76	-	-
Exclusive	0.88	-	-
Leisure	-	0.89	-
Sports	-	0.87	-
Music	-	0.87	-
Metaphysical	0.82	0.87	-
Death	0.82	-	-
Physical	-0.72	-	-
Body	-0.79	-	-
Sexual	-	0.75	-
Eating	-0.72	-	-
Sleep	-0.81	-	-
Swear	-	0.81	-

6.3 Discussion

There are several themes that are present or implied in both the computer and qualitative analyses.

- An increase in suicidal thoughts and focus on death over time
- An ongoing debate regarding the pros and cons of living versus ending his life
- An increased awareness that he is writing for an audience
- A desire to communicate the reasons for taking his life – in particular, that it is not the alcohol but rather life-long low self-esteem and "laziness"
- Indications of stress and depression are highest in the middle of the journal and decline toward the end
- Jim is a master of denial and escape – his writing details his activity with television shows and movies, music and computer games, as well as diet and food preparations and drinks
- The LIWC analysis identified an increase in positive emotions over the course of the diary, which replicates the trend observed in Katie's diary (Chapter 3).

Jim was very different when sober for a week – energetic and moving in a more positive direction. But he did not see this. This change was not salient for him. It was not reinforcing for him. Why not? Jim was depressed. He rarely used that word in his writing (which is perhaps characteristic of men) but the symptoms are there – sadness, irritability, tension, lack of motivation, feelings of worthlessness and hopelessness, suicidal thoughts. As an escape from the depression, he drinks (characteristic of men) and uses escapist activities (television and computer games)

Jim was bright, inquisitive, analytical and technologically skilled, but he did not acknowledge these strengths. Jim was a good person with a sense of ethics. For example, he would not cash a bad check, and he called his bank to apologize for being angry at them. Although Jim avoided the intervention that his family had planned for him, later, just prior to his death, he fantasized that someone might call or stop by to intervene and wondered whether he should call his sister or a good friend

Jim vacillated about dying. He planned it for certain days, but those days passed without his taking his own life. It seems that he dealt with this vacillation by "painting himself into a corner" in which suicide was the only option. He had no money left, his utilities were being shut off (including his Internet access and telephone), and his would probably lose his house.

Whereas in other diaries, such as Katie's Diary (see Chapter 3 above), the suicide comes as a surprise (Katie sounded better, more positive and stronger toward the end), Jim's suicide seems more likely as the final nine weeks and nine days pass.

6.4 Jim's Sister

For this diary, there is an extra source of data. We asked Jim's sister who was both brave and kind to give us the diary for our research. What did she expect from our study, and what are her thoughts on her brother?

David: What were your motives in giving me the diary? What did you hope or expect?
Judy: Those are good questions. I'll try to answer as best I can. My desire and motivation in giving you the diary started with meeting and working with Donna Barnes. I found it interesting that there were people who actually study the writings of people who ultimately die by suicide and at the same time these writings are relatively scarce. I was holding volumes of writings from my brother prior to his suicide where he recorded both mundane daily activities and thoughts about his imminent suicide and his actual decision-making process as he struggled as to decide whether to call me or to proceed with his suicide plans. I feel fortunate to have access to what was going on in his head about his life and why he decided to end his life. Many suicide survivors are caught completely by surprise and have no clue as to why their loved ones died by suicide.

Ultimately, I think my hope is for a small sense of purpose if Jim's writing somehow adds to the body of knowledge about suicide and why people choose suicide. Somewhere in his diary, Jim states that maybe his ramblings might help someone else. Although I think he was referring to his alcohol dependence, I think he would feel good that, even if he couldn't save himself, he might help someone else.

I've developed a predictable interest in the subject of suicide from an academic perspective. I have a lot of curiosity about what the diary reveals to an emotionally neutral academic study. I knew Jim well and, by reading everything he wrote, I feel like I know even more about him. Some people thought he had an agenda in his writing, but I know he did not; he just wrote straight up what was going through his head. I'm interested in knowing how his pre-suicide writing compares to others you have studied.

David: I am now writing up a brief scholarly paper based on Jim's diary. What are your thoughts and feelings as you await this? What do you expect to think and feel after reading it?

Judy: As far as what I'd feel after reading your paper, thinking about his diary always brings some sadness, but four years has given me emotional distance. My intellectual curiosity and academic interest in the subject is compartmentalized differently than my emotions (if that makes sense).

David: I have one more question. If you were writing a scholarly article on Jim's suicide–like a case study–what factors would you focus on?

Judy: I have been giving this a lot of thought and I have come up with several things that I would focus on, this after going through the exercise of searching on the word "kill" in the diary. I cut and pasted all the entries about Jim's questioning about killing himself. Putting them all together makes me think that the frequency of writing about killing himself increases: Feb – 2; Mar – 2; Apr – 1; May – 10; June – 14; July – 10; Aug–11. The process of "should I or should I not" and "can I or can I not" goes on for over seven months. Toward the later part of the diary, he narrows his options down to (1) kill myself, and (2) call Judy. "Call Judy" is an "out." He didn't believe he could turn his life around himself, so one option was to turn his life over for someone else to put his life back together for him. The way he describes the severity of the pain seems to be more intense over time, as well as the deterioration of his physical health.

Low or lack of self esteem is a core factor in his suicide. He suffered from depression (genetic, the entire family does). Previous handwritten diaries show him going through periods of trying self-improvement activities (and always failing at them).

Alcoholism is a strong factor, although he insisted that laziness was more of a factor than the alcohol. I'm not positive about this, and would have to study more – I don't think his alcohol consumption increased as he got closer to his death.

One other strong factor is his family and parents and not feeling loved. Our parents definitely lacked any kind of parenting skills. The best example I can give of this is on the day of "Joe's eye accident." The two boys (roughly 5 and 8) were playing and tossing stuffed animals down the stairs. Joe was at the bottom. One animal hit and dislodged a suspended ceiling panel and the metal framework that holds them in place. The metal hit Joe in the eye, cutting it severely. My grandmother was babysitting the boys at the time, and she didn't know enough to call anyone. Joe was screaming in pain until our mother got home and took him to the ER. (Joe ended up blind in that eye). Jim was left to witness Joe's screaming in pain. Afterwards, Jim was blamed, yelled at by Dad, and "threatened" by Dad according to Jim's diary entry. No one comforted Jim and assured him that it wasn't his fault, or talked to Jim at all about it, except for yelling, blaming and threatening. All that being said, more information, recollections from siblings would be needed to develop this aspect of Jim's suicide contributors.

6.5 Final Comment

In this analysis of Jim's diary, we used three approaches: a qualitative analysis by a skilled psychologist, the LIWC analysis, and the thoughts from Jim's sister. The thoughts from Jim's sister are based on Jim's complete life story and are, therefore, based on different information. The qualitative analysis and the LIWC analysis are based on only what is in the diary, and so the conclusions are more limited. However, this triangulation provides a richer understanding of Jim and the motivations behind his choice of suicide than either approach alone.

7 A Suicide in Academia[25]

Robert was an Assistant Professor in the humanities at a major university in the Midwest of America. He had served two years in the military and had explored a career in the arts before going back to university to earn a Ph.D. He had had two temporary teaching positions at the instructor level before obtaining a tenure track position at a major research-oriented university. He was married and, at the beginning of the diary, he and his wife had just welcomed a son.

The diary starts with a couple of entries in 1931, two entries in 1932, and begins in earnest in August 1933. There follow 71 entries up to October 1935. He died by suicide in July 1936.

7.1 Robert's Relationship with his Parents

At the beginning of the diary, Robert had been in psychoanalytically-oriented psychotherapy, and he found it useful. He was persuaded of the validity of psychoanalytic theory and its applicability to his life. He became particularly concerned about his possible incestuous desires toward his mother, the rivalry with his father, and the competition with his brothers, especially his younger siblings, for the attention of his mother.

> In other words, I was never mother-weaned. I am fixated at an early stage of development. And I continue to react in infantile ways based on infantile emotions.

Later that day, he wrote:

> I don't want to, but I am going to force myself to say that today I felt ugly and dirty and ashamed. Recognizing, or beginning to recognize my incest (I can't even write it right) tendencies brings down on my Ego the Super-ego wrath (i.e., feelings of dirtiness, filth, scumminess, unworthiness.....)

In the context of his present life, he saw the parallel of these childhood concerns with the competition he felt toward his newborn son for the attention of his wife. As a new member of the department, hoping for tenure even though it was clear at the beginning that tenure was unlikely (he realized this in March 1934 after talking with a senior member of the department[26]), he saw the competition with the other new

25 I have taken great care to disguise the details of "Robert" to ensure that it is impossible to identify the real individual.

26 In high prestige universities in those years, Assistant Professors rarely received tenure. After working for five years, they were expected to move elsewhere, continue to improve their scholarly record and then, perhaps, be rehired at a senior level.

members of the department as similar to the earlier rivalry with his siblings. He even equated the prestigious university with his mother, calling it "Mother X," so that the fear of reappointment for Robert was a reminder of his mother rejecting him in favor of his younger siblings.

All this may have been true, but the insight does not seem to have allayed his anxieties and anger. Rather, it gave him material on which to ruminate in his diary. It is difficult to evaluate rumination in diaries. If we were to write down every thought we had in the course of a day, week or month about an issue that bothers us, we too might seem to be ruminating. The fact that these thoughts are written down and take up many pages perhaps leads the reader to perceive rumination whereas the preoccupation with the issue may be no more than that which occupies our unwritten thoughts. Nevertheless, many pages of this diary are concerned with repeated examination of these issues with his mother and siblings, his wife and son, and his colleagues.

Since he views his wife as a mother substitute, he feels inhibited when anticipating sexual intercourse, and he deals with this by drinking, often "fast" to use his own words. However, his wife is often repelled by his tipsiness. He also fears that his wife has a poor opinion of him.

> ...I can *never* really please her really, that she sneers at me behind my back, that she views me as a feminine and weak and helpless character, that she laughs when I fail, and laughs when I succeed because she thinks I'm kidding about my successes, that ("again" she *tolerates* me, that she is "putting up" with me 'til something better comes along, that I'm no good really and I can't prove to her (or anyone else) that I am, that I'm a poor schnook in her eyes, that I'm to be pitied.....

Sex is full of conflict for Robert. "Last night, [his wife] came into my study and said in effect, "come to bed with me." I was reluctant, yet eager.....I seem to have a perpetual conflict re: sex: (a) I want to dictate it, and (b) I want [my wife] to request it." After they have sex, Robert does not want to sleep in the bed with his wife "Because we've done something that is bad.?"

His father also causes him conflict.

> I am a better man, in terms of achievement.....than he ever was....I want the scalp in my hand, as it were. But more important, I feel horribly guilty and anxiety ridden for outdoing him.

7.2 Interpersonal Relationships

Robert had interpersonal difficulties. His was inhibited in his speech, and he had difficulty with watering eyes, which he calls crying but which may have been no more than allergies. When he refers to his eyes, he never uses words such as sobbing, although at times he mentions that they water a lot. "I tend to cry (my nose is always stopped up and my eyes water), I flush or blush all the time." He writes that he must improve in his social interactions.

He writes frequently throughout the diary that he is lonely. "I have no friends to console me – I've never been able to make friends." "I feel now, as I did long ago, that I'm alone and rejected." His relationships with intimates is also colored by his fear that they will use him.

> i.e., when a woman indicates interest in me, particularly of a sexual nature, I tend to retreat, feeling that she doesn't mean it, that she is trying to "get something from me," that she will "use me to her own advantage."

7.3 Work

Robert was also full of fear and anxiety, both in class and in the department and committee meetings. Fear and anxiety is normal for a new instructor. It is difficult to decide how forceful to be in meetings. Too little participation and too forceful participation may both hinder chances of promotion and tenure. Preparing lectures in the first year of a job is time-consuming – indeed one sometimes fails to prepare enough material to finish a class. Later on, one often realizes that one's lecture notes are woefully inadequate, and they have to be re-done.

At the same time, being at a major research-oriented university, Robert also had to publish. He managed to do this and produced a dozen papers during the four years that he was at the university, all in the best journals in his field. But, not atypically, there were periods when he had trouble writing, and these times concerned him. He worked hard, but feared that his contributions would be overlooked. He also saw success as a lose-lose situation: ".....if I do a good job, I'll be punished, and if I do a bad one, I'll be discarded. What a hell of a conflict to be in."

7.4 An Impostor

His scholarly work was impeded by his fear that he was a fraud – an impostor. This extended to all spheres:

> .....my fears are very real, i.e., they are very *strong*. And, as I continue to think about the problem, they do center about the problem of yielding, of being controlled; and even more important, of being ridiculed and laughed at. The latter is important in all phases of my life, my endeavors: teaching, research, writing, sex, interpersonal relations......

When he gives a talk at a conference that is received well by his audience, he is reassured, but only temporarily.

> This experience has left me with *less* of the feeling that I am a useless cog in society, that I don't count, that no one cares what I do, that my actions are fruitless, that I'm stupid and incapable, that I should have entered another profession, that my case is hopeless....that I'm not a blot on the societal world, a misfit, a cancer, a sponger, a misnomer, etc....If you tell me in whatever way that I am not worthless, you are fooling me – you are kidding – you don't really mean it.

What is interesting in this part of the entry is that Robert moves from mentioning the accolades he received to stating the feeling of being an impostor in its strongest terms. He calls himself a cancer, and he sees others are kidding him when they imply that he is not worthless. Because he sees others as laughing at him, he rages against them.

> It's no wonder I tend to cry, currently, when I am earnestly engaged in face-to-face contacts with my professional colleagues. These are literally tears of frustration, i.e., "I'm doing the best I can, but you are laughing at me – I can't strike you, all I can do is to cry in helpless frustration." And roughly the same with my students: "I'm pouring out my knowledge to you, the fruits of the sweat of my brow – and you are secretly laughing; I can't slay you, all I can do is to cry in helpless frustration.

Yet at times, he realizes that he is a good scholar, a good teacher, and a good committee chair. His articles are published in the best journals, his student evaluation of teaching scores are solid, and he successfully restructures the courses offered by his department one by one.

7.5 Paranoia

Related to Robert's feeling that he is a fraud is his paranoia. On four occasions in the diary, he expresses a fear that the FBI will obtain his diary and prosecute him for it. I see nothing in it that would have any interest for the FBI or that would lead to any criminal charges. "I am basically paranoid, yet afraid to be too much so outwardly although my actions must show it." Robert says that his father had paranoid tendencies too. "I feel persecuted. I have my dad's paranoiac tendencies." "After all, my father had real paranoid tendencies, and these I learned from him. During the recent present I have become aware of my own 'persecution' tendencies which I now perceive to be traceable directly to my father." The feelings of persecution are particularly relevant to his sexual thoughts. "And I also feel as though everyone present *knows what I am thinking*! This is unrealistic, but terribly painful." His paranoia extends to his wife.

> .....she wants intercourse, she wants me to kowtow, to take advantage of me, so that she can laugh behind my back at my ineptitude.....And, best of all, she wants to humiliate me, to make me appear ridiculous.....And so I'll have to be circumspect and very careful – else.....she will report my ludicrous behavior to "him" – others – and they will have gay sport over it.

Robert appears to realize that his bizarre thoughts are not grounded in reality, and so he does not appear to be psychotic. In March 1935, when he writes of feeling exploited, he says: "By the way, this is in all probability not true – the important thing at the moment is that I feel that it is true." Yet he does fear becoming mad, although he confuses multiple personality with schizophrenia, a common error in those not informed about psychology.

> And besides, I have been feeling that there are at least "two of me" – the outward behaving one and the inward feeling one! (The first signs of schizophrenia?)

Robert also perceives an inner conflict: intense rage generated by any signs of disapproval by his superiors and intense fear generated by these rage states. Over the years, he turned more and more to alcohol as his fear reducer, which added to his marital conflicts since his wife disapproved of his excessive drinking.

His psychological state was made worse by the prospective birth of a second child, a prospect that he dreaded. He did not want a second rival for his wife's affection and attention. However, this son was born severely defective and immediately placed in an institution. This led Robert to feel guilty over his death wishes for this child. The child was born in November 1934, and, two days later, Robert wrote that he was narrowly averting a nervous breakdown. Only alcohol helped.

7.6 Merging Work and Sex

On several occasions during the diary, Robert talks of problems and conflicts over work and immediately moves to problems and conflicts with sex. In my discussion of the diary of Cesare Pavese (Chapter 4 above), the Italian novelist who killed himself, I noted the reverse tendency – that Pavese's failure in love led him to disparage his work. For Robert, the sequence moves in the opposite direction.

> .....I was brought to [the university] as a joke......A great joke, he's nothing but a small town jerk. And it's time he found it out. My father used to criticize me all the time. It was his way of "getting even" with me.....But wherein lies the shameful feelings I have? Sex, no doubt. Things I do for my own pleasure or gratification are shameful

This is written in the space of ten lines of text.

In writing of a seminar that he has been invited to attend, he feels that it is beneath him – that he is superior to the other participants. "I don't need the affiliation with these men, at least one of whom I consider stupid." Five lines later he writes: "What is it? I'm afraid I am going too fast – that I can't back up my public wares. Beyond that feeling is sex: I am going far too fast! (i.e., too many intercourses [per unit time] scares me)" In a later entry, Robert writes, "If I could only learn that my professional activities are not sexual in nature *per se*." This sequence has been called a maladaptive cognitive structure by Kovacs and Beck (1978) where one thought leads to another, creating a more potent cognitive distortion.

7.7 Suicide

The first mention of suicide in the diary occurs in January 1935.

> So, what can I do about it all? I can "suppress" the problem by immersing myself in work (as I do). I can "drown" the problem in alcohol, as I've been doing. I can "face" the problem, even though I've defined it very inadequately. I can run away in a literal sense (suicide, going away, etc.). I can ignore the problem and go on suffering. I can work on it through self-analysis.

Later he writes that he thought of suicide as a child. "I remember looking out of my childhood living room window at the rain, the snow, the bare and stark wintry apple trees blowing in the wind, and thinking that suicide is the only answer." ".....staring out the windows at the rain when I was a kid and wishing I was dead." In the same diary entry as this last quote, in March 1935, Robert wrote "Several times tonight the thought of suicide has crossed my mind, as it did when I was a small child and felt completely rejected by my parents. A way out – almost any way out – that is what I want."

7.8 The End

Toward the end of Robert's life, the entries in the diary become less frequent. In February 1935, he developed skin eruptions, and his dermatologist told him that the causes were emotional which Robert interpreted as meaning a result of his incestuous desires. That same month, he attributed his blushing to his having forbidden thoughts, "i.e., that I am recognizing directly my attraction to [his wife] (à la Mom), and reacting viscerally, with shame, to such recognition." In October 1935, as the decision of tenure comes closer, he is back in psychotherapy, a decision that his wife had been urging for some time.[27] He reports that he has been having panic attacks and managed to see a psychiatrist, just in time, who gave him medication and emergency psychotherapy. He mentions that he almost fainted in the first session from fear and, when he was told in the second session that he had a neurosis, he broke down in tears.

---

27 One night in March that year, when he tried to talk to her about his problems, she told him to grow up.

In the next, final entry, in May 1936, Robert reports that he is still having panic attacks and has the foreboding that disaster is just around the corner. He is afraid of his wife and his colleagues. He is spending hours in bed, smoking, and drinking. He mentions that he is on his fourth quart at the time of writing this entry. He looks at his hands, and the last words in his diary are:

> They are currently non-productive. This is just about as discouraging to me as my "idea" mal-productions! Ambition is present – with no real outlet. Please give me, guide me to the outlet!!!

He killed himself six weeks later.

7.9 Discussion

It is hard to understand the psychodynamics of suicide from suicide notes and yet, although the information provided by the diary of a suicide is richer, we are still left with many unanswered questions. From Robert's diary we gain a phenomenological understanding of the conflicts that preceded and, perhaps, resulted in his decision to kill himself. What is missing, however, is an understanding of how these conflicts developed in him. What childhood experiences and trauma led to his conflicts. For example, given that Robert seems convinced of the Oedipal bases for the problems with his wife and in academia, did his parents behave in a way as to exacerbate his Oedipal conflicts? We do not know. The same is true for his feelings of being a sham and a fraud, for his paranoia, and so on.

However, we are able to identify many of the conflicts with which Robert was faced. Indeed, his life is full of lose-lose situations, with no win-win situations. He wants intimacy with his wife, feels rejected if she refuses, yet he fears ridicule from her and experiences guilt if she agrees. He wants to publish good scholarly work, but worries whether his work is being accepted merely so that his peers can attack him and criticize him after it appears. He wants to be seen as competent in departmental matters at work, but worries that he will be punished in some way for being competent.

The psychotherapy that he received on two occasions, before the diary commences and at the end of his life, may have helped him cope, but it also appears to have given fodder for his anxiety disorder. Rather than the possible insights giving him an understanding of the root of some of his problems and calming him, they appear to have given him issues to worry about and ruminate over. Was psychoanalytic-oriented psychotherapy the best approach for such an individual, or would a more cognitive-behavioral approach (not available at the time) have worked better?[28] I discussed the role of rumination in Chapter 3 on Katie, and the same discussion applies here. Did writing the diary and ruminating on his possible Oedipal conflicts help or harm Robert?

In the diaries that have been explored hitherto, both those of ordinary individuals and those of famous people, it has been impossible to obtain the clinical records (especially from psychotherapists) to provide an alternative interpretation of the person. Should this ever be possible, it would enrich our understanding of the suicidal mind.

7.10 The LIWC Analysis

The entries in Robert's diary were analyzed by the LIWC program, both over the whole length of the diary (for four years, numbered 1-75) and for the entries in the final year (numbered 1-53).

Over the whole length of the diary, Robert showed much more concern with himself. Negative emotions increased in frequency, including sadness. He focused more the present as time passed, became less interested in causation, and showed more concern with his body (including sexual and eating activities). He also swore more. In the last year of the diary, most of these same trends were also present, including a greater concern with himself and less concern with his family. Both positive and negative emotions showed a tendency to decline, and there was less mention of death. The decline in mentions of death over the course of the final year is in accord with Spiegel and Neuringer's (1963) prediction that, as individuals approach the time of their suicidal action, they will mention words associated with death and suicide less.

It can be seen that the changes in emotions do not parallel the trends seen in the previous diaries examined in this book (except for the tendency for a decline in negative emotions). On the whole, Robert's mental state worsened over time. Whereas readers of Katie's diary thought that she sounded stronger toward the end of the diary, Robert is clearly disintegrating, and so his suicide is not unexpected.

28 At the time that this was taking place, psychoanalytic psychotherapy was the major form of counseling available.

Tab. 7.1: Correlations over time in Robert's diary

	May, Year 1 to October, Year 5: numbered 1-75	**Final Year numbered 1-53**
	Pearson r	Pearson r
Words longer than 6 letters	-0.40**	-0.42**
Pronouns	0.42**	0.28*
First person singular	0.42**	0.26#
Total first person	0.43**	0.31*
Negations	0.35**	0.37**
Numbers	-0.28*	-0.05
Positive feelings	-0.01	-0.24#
Negative emotions	0.22#	-0.26#
Anger	0.13	-0.31*
Sad	0.22#	0.04
Causation	-0.27*	-0.29*
Insight	-0.15	-0.23#
Discrepancies	0.24*	0.11
Senses	0.27*	0.20
Feeling	0.30**	0.06
Communication	-0.25*	0.04
Family	0.08	-0.38**
Present tense verbs	0.32**	0.26#
Down	0.24*	0.44**
Job	-0.10	0.26#
Sports	0.20#	0.20
TV	0.20#	0.22
Death	0.08	-0.28*
Physical states	0.31**	0.11
Sexual	0.33**	0.08
Eating	0.22#	0.29*
Swear	0.39**	0.30*

* two-tailed $p < .05$, ** two-tailed $p < .01$, # trend (two-tailed $p < .10$)

8 The Diary of Kenneth Williams[29]

Kenneth Williams (1926-1988) was born in London, the son of a barber. He was educated at Lyulph Stanley School, became an apprentice draughtsman to a mapmaker and joined the army in 1944. He first performed on stage while in the Royal Engineers. In 1948 he began acting in repertory theater but failed to become a serious dramatic actor. A producer for the radio saw him on the stage in Bernard Shaw's *St Joan* in 1954 and saw his potential as a comic performer. He appeared on the radio series *Hancock's Half Hour* for five years and moved on to other radio comedy shows. He appeared in several West End revues with, among others, Maggie Smith and Fenella Fielding. In the 1960s and 1970s, he starred in the British film series *Carry On* which were very successful but for which the actors were paid poorly. In his diaries, Williams was critical of the series and of his own performances in the films. As he grew older, he appeared on the BBC radiio panel game *Just a Minute*, contributed to *What's My Line*, and hosted *International Cabaret*.

Hia father died in 1962 after drinking posion (carbon tetracholride), a death that was ruled accidental, but for which Scotland Yard considered Williams a possible murder suspect. Williams seems to have been celibate, certainly from his 40s on, and his diaries imply that he had homosexual inclinations. Since homosexuality was a crime in England up until 1967, Williams seems to have suppressed these desires as much as he could and contented himself with masturbation.[30]

Williams lived in a series of small rented apartments in London from the mid-1950s until his death. After his father died, Williams's mother moved into an apartment next door, and Williams spent a lot of time (albeit with some friction) with her. Williams wrote of his loneliness, despondency and sense of underachievement and, in his last few years, his depressions worsened as his health declined. He killed himself on April 15, 1988, with an overdose of barbiturates. Although the official verdict was an "open verdict," English coroners are well-known for covering up suicides (Lester 2002a), and Williams's death was certainly suicide.

The last year of Williams's diary (Davies, 1993) , from April 15, 1987, to April 14, 1988, was analyzed using the LIWC. Pearson correlations coefficients were calculated between the content scores from the LIWC and number of the entry for the last year (167 entries, numbered 1-167), the last month (30 entries, numbered 1-30) and the last week (7 entries, numbered 1-7) of Williams's life (see Table 8-1).

---

29 This chapter was written by John F. Gunn IIII and David Lester

30 Williams accompanied the gay couple Joe Orton and Kenneth Halliwell to Morocco for holidays, a common place for gay men in England to travel for casual sex with local boys.

8.1 The Last Year

For the last year of Williams's diary, ten significant associations were found. There was an increase in the number of words in each entry, but a decrease in the uniqueness of the words and in the percentage of words longer than six letters. Williams also made more references to time. There was a significant decrease in references to occupation and jobs. Finally there was a significant increase in references made to grooming.

Tab. 8.1: Analyses over time (entries) of the diary of Kenneth Williams

	Last year n=167 numbered 1-167	Last month n=30 numbered 1-30	Last week n=7 numbered 1-7
Word count	0.54**	0.40*	-0.10
Unique words	-0.48**	-0.38*	-0.02
Words longer than 6 letters	-0.20*	-0.44*	-0.15
Negations	0.03	0.04	0.68#
Prepositions	0.14#	-0.14	-0.37
Numbers	0.14#	-0.05	0.06
Positive feelings	-0.15#	0.07	-0.80
Discrepancies	0.15#	-0.03	-0.54
Social processes	-0.11	-0.03	-0.84*
Friends	-0.13#	0.10	-
Family	-0.07	0.31#	-0.30
Time	0.23**	0.28	-0.10
Past tense verbs	0.15#	0.19	0.12
Space	0.04	0.15	-0.69#
Down	0.14#	-0.01	-0.25
Inclusive	-0.16*	-0.17	-0.10
Occupations	-0.18*	-0.30	0.13
Job	-0.18	-0.24	0.16
Money	-0.06	0.42*	0.34
Metaphysical	0.06	-0.10	-0.69#
Death	0.02	-0.08	-0.82*
Grooming	0.24**	-0.12	0.20

* two-tailed $p < .05$, ** two-tailed $p < .01$, # trend (two-tailed $p < .10$)

8.2 The Last Month

For the last month of Williams's diary only four significant relationships were found. As with the last year of the diary, the last month showed an increase in the number of words, but a decrease in the proportion of unique words and in the percentage of words longer than six letters. Finally there was an increase in references to money.

8.3 The Last Week

For the last week of Williams's diary, there were only three significant relationships. There was a decrease in positive feelings, a decrease in reference to social processes, and a decrease in references to death.

8.4 Discussion

Unlike the findings in Chapter 3, in which the diary of a young girl was analyzed, and Chapter 4, in which the last year of Cesare Pavese's diary was analyzed, this study did not find a statistically significant increase in the percentage of positive emotions as the entries got closer to the time of the suicide. There was an increase in positive feelings in the final week of his diary, but the final week only had seven diary entries to analyze. This lack of significance for positive emotions overall could be related to the fact that Kenneth Williams suffered from recurring ulcers and back pain which was a repeated topic in later entries.

As shown by the increase in word count found in both the analysis of the last year and the analysis of the last month of Williams's diary, his entries did increase in length. This increase in length however, was countered by a decrease in the overall sophistication of the writing. His entries got longer, but the words became shorter and less unique. In an analysis of Van Gogh's letters to his sisters (Chapter 16), I found that there was also a decrease in the percentage of longer words.

Finally in the last week of his life there was a decrease in references to social processes and death. This can be seen as a turning inward and perhaps a focus more on himself the closer he got to the time of his suicide, and also the dwindling of his social role. The decrease in references to death supports the hypothesis of Spiegel and Neuringer (1963) who predicted that, prior to the suicidal act, a person's thinking may be diverted from thoughts of death. However, overall, the LIWC analysis of Williams's diary provides fewer psychodynamic insights than the analyses in earlier chapters.

9 Wallace Baker

Wallace Baker killed himself by drowning off Manhattan Beach in New York on September 28, 1913. He sent a diary to the editor of a magazine before he died who forwarded the diary to a literary magazine, *The Glebe*, which published ten issues in 1913 and 1914. This magazine published the diary in the October issue of 1913 (Baker, 1913).[31] Cavan (1965) discussed this diary.

The diary consists of 40 entries written over a period of 19 months, and the last entry was made on the day of Wallace Baker's suicide. Baker was a young man (23 years old when he killed himself) who seems to have been relatively uneducated, but who considered himself to be a possible genius. He had literary interests and read the great novelists, playwrights and philosophers, such as Ibsen and Nietzsche. However, he does not seem to have written anything besides his diary. He was unable to afford to go to college. He worked in secretarial jobs and was consumed by his sexual appetite. Having no partner, he frequently visited prostitutes and then felt disgusted with himself afterwards.

Baker described himself quite succinctly in an entry on September 1, 1912.

> ....I am doing my best in a sincere manner under the circumstances, namely, that I must go through life with health impaired to a greater or lesser extent; that I am inclined to extremes, pessimistic or very cheerful, even childish, by turns; that life appeals to me when I think as terribly inevitable that I have a tendency to degeneracy at times (which I feel I can overcome to a certain extent by heroic measures); that the happiness of a home and children of my own may be denied me. (p. 51)

Cavan viewed Baker as introspective and egocentric in a typically adolescent way. He had hardly any friends outside of his family. His two goals in life were to become an author and to be sexual continent. In reality, his sexual desires may have by normal but, lacking any partner, he began to visit prostitutes. He wrote on several occasions that free love should become the norm and that men and women should be free to have sex with whomever they desired. His inability to form mature relationships with peers and his disgust over sex with prostitutes raises unanswered questions about the way he was raised by his parents and the values that they instilled in him.

Cavan felt that Baker's diary gives little evidence of writing ability. He tried to write, but Cavan concluded that he found himself with little to write about. His writing remained a grandiose dream, although he admitted to occasional doubts in the diary. Typically, however, he blamed his failure to produce any good writing on external factors, such as lack of money and poor health.

Eventually, Baker began to worry that he was becoming insane. Suicide seems to have always been in his mind, and one wonders whether psychiatric disorder and

31 This magazine was reproduced by Kraus Reprints (New York) in 1967.

suicide ran in his family. Baker's despair and hopelessness seems to have increased leading up to his suicide, and the last entry, written on the day of his death, is his suicide note.

9.1 The LIWC Analysis

Only seven significant associations were identified and nine trends out of the 74 associations examined (see Table 9-1). Of psychological interest, anxiety seemed to decrease over time, but concern with death increased. References to achievement increased, as did concern with work (and occupation and jobs). Concerns with the body (and sleep) decreased.

Tab. 9.1: Correlations over time for the 40 entries in Wallace Baker's diary

	Over entry (1-40)	**Over day of the entry from the beginning of diary (0-673)**
Emoticons	-0.27#	-0.23
Negations	0.32*	0.27#
Article	-0.32*	-0.30#
Anxiety	-0.28#	-0.22
Certainty	-0.27#	-0.28#
Senses	0.24	0.28#
Hearing	0.40**	0.42**
Communication	0.29#	0.30#
Occupations	0.29#	0.28#
Job	0.30#	0.31#
Achievement	0.53***	0.51***
Leisure	0.31*	0.27#
Home	0.27#	0.19
Death	0.28#	0.33*
Body	-0.29#	-0.29#
Sleep	-0.40*	-0.37*

* two-tailed p < .05, * two-tailed p < .05, ** two-tailed p < .01, *** two-tailed p < .001, # trend (two-tailed p < .10)

A reading of the diary perhaps resolves these conflicting trends. As time passed, his concern with achievement (in his case, becoming a brilliant author) and the low level job that he had, associated with the trends toward more negations (such as not and never) and less certainty (such as always and never) suggests that his belief in his ability to achieve his goals declined and that death became a more probable alternative to failure.

10 Bobby Sands[32]

Bobby Sands was a member of the Irish Republican Army in Northern Ireland and was imprisoned by the British courts for his activities. He went on hunger strike while in prison and died in H Block of HMP Maze (Long Kesh) prison on May 5th 1981 at the age of 27. Bobby Sands was born in 1954 in Rathcode, a predominantly loyalist district of north Belfast. As a result of his final arrest and imprisonment, he was sentenced in September 1977 to fourteen years. He was denied the category of "political prisoner" and imprisoned instead as an "ordinary prisoner." The prisoners so labeled protested this action in various ways (such as refusing to wear the prison uniform), until some of the prisoners decided to go on a hunger strike. The second hunger strike started on March 1st 1981, and Bobby Sands died on the 66th day of his hunger strike, on May 5th. He kept a diary for the first 17 days of his hunger strike (Sands, 1998), and the present study analyzed his diary using the LIWC program.

Two points must be made here. Bobby Sands did not die in the same way as the other individuals discussed in this section. His goal was not to die, but rather to protest the treatment of IRA prisoners by the British courts. However, he was aware that his death was possible, if not likely, and his actions did indeed result in his death. Whether martyrs are "suicides" or not is a matter of debate which illustrates the absence of a good nomenclature for labeling self-induced deaths.

Second, the diary of Bobby Sands diary ends before his death. This was true of Katie's diary also, although her diary ended only ten days before her death. Researchers may wonder how the content of the diary might have changed had it extended up to the day of death but, in the cases of Katie and Bobby Sands, we cannot know.

10.1 The LIWC Analysis

The 17 entries in the diary of Bobby Sands were analyzed by the LIWC program. The entries were numbered from 1 to 17, and Pearson correlation coefficients were calculated between the entry number and each of the 74 content variables in order to identify linear trends over the 17 days. The results are shown in Table 10-1. Of the 74 variables examined, six correlation coefficients were statistically significant, and a further seven were close to statistical significance.

In the earlier study of Katie's diary, Pennbaker and Stone (2004) found an increase in positive emotions as the day of Katie's death came closer. The same increase in positive emotions was found in the diary of Bobby Sands, as well as an increase in positive feelings. As with Katie's diary, there was a decrease in words concerned with death over time in the diary of Bobby Sands. This result is consistent with the study

32 I would like to thank John Connolly for stimulating this chapter and for buying the published diary for me.

Tab. 10.1: Correlations over the last 17 days of Bobby Sands' life (numbered 1-17)

	Pearson r
Total second person	0.45#
Articles	0.47#
Prepositions	0.45#
Numbers	-0.48*
Positive emotions	0.54*
Positive feelings	0.48#
Cognitive processes	-0.43#
Inhibition	-0.65**
Seeing	0.41#
Metaphysical issues	-0.52*
Religion	-0.47#
Death	-0.45#
Physical states	0.49*
Eating	0.75**

* two-tailed p < .05, ** two-tailed p < .01, # trend (two-tailed p < .10)

by Spiegel and Neuringer (1963), which I have cited many times already in this book, who speculated that the suicide notes of completed suicides would avoid mentioning words associated with death and suicide since there would be tendency to avoid thinking of the act they were about to choose. In a comparison of genuine and simulated suicide notes, the genuine notes did have fewer mentions of suicide. The diaries of both Katie and Bobby Sands had a decline in death-related words over time as the time of their death came closer.

As the diary of Bobby Sands progressed, there was an increase in concern with his physical state and with eating, as might be expected in someone who was engaged in a hunger strike. Some of the changes identified in Katie's diary (changes in personal pronouns, social words, negative emotions, and question marks) were not found in the diary of Bobby Sands. In addition, whereas there was an increase in religious words over time in Katie's diary, religious words declined over time in the diary of Bobby Sands.

Several unique findings were identified in the diary of Bobby Sands over time. There were decreases in words concerned with metaphysical issues and with inhibition (such as "block" and "constraint") and a trend toward fewer words concerned with cognitive processes (such as "cause" and "know").

The results of this analysis of the diary of Bobby Sands during his hunger strike that resulted in his death show some similarities to previous studies of the diary of a young woman who died by suicide, but also some differences. The differences are to be expected since, not only was the intent of Bobby Sands not to kill himself but rather to make a political protest, but also because each individual is unique in the psychodynamics of their behavior.

Part II: **Studies of Suicide Notes**

11 The Study of Genuine and Simulated Notes

Shneidman and Farberow (1957b) published a sample of suicide notes that they found in the files of the Los Angeles medical examiner's office. They matched the 33 genuine suicide notes with 33 "simulated" suicide notes, that is, suicide notes solicited from people who were not contemplating suicide who were asked to pretend that they were going to complete suicide and to write a suicide note. Since then, many papers have appeared comparing this set of genuine and simulated suicide notes.[33]

Lester (1988a) has argued that this comparison does not shed light on the mind of suicidal individuals but rather examines whether nonsuicidal individuals have any insight into the suicidal mind. Since many studies have found differences between the genuine and the simulated suicide notes, the evidence is that nonsuicidal individuals do not have good insights into the suicidal mind. For example, a small proportion (15%) of the genuine suicide notes in Shneidman and Farberow's sample have anger in them directed toward a significant other, while none of the simulated suicide notes do so (Lester, 1989c). All this tells us is that nonsuicidal individuals do not realize that a small proportion of suicidal individuals are angry.

Instead, Lester suggested that simulated suicide notes are a good way to study the *opinions* and *myths* that people in the general population have about suicides and suicidal behavior. For example, in his sample of simulated notes, Lester found that women more often addressed their simulated suicide note to someone than did the men, apologized and asked forgiveness, stated that they were unhappy, and said that others would be better off if they were dead. Thus, men and woman appear to have different conceptions about the motives for suicide.

What might make a better comparison group for genuine suicide notes? Ideally, we need letters and notes written by these suicides at an earlier time when they were not suicidal. Then we could see how their psychological state had changed from the nonsuicidal period to the suicidal period. Unfortunately, most individuals do not have collections of letters and notes written over the course of their lifetime. Furthermore, regrettable though it is, researchers are sometimes lazy. It is easy to collect a sample of simulated suicide notes. For example, Shneidman and Farberow went to labor unions and fraternal groups and asked groups of men to write simulated suicide notes. I have asked students in my courses on suicide to write such notes. A captive group of people can write simulated suicide notes in ten minutes. To collect earlier letters from deceased suicides requires tracing the significant others of each suicide, visiting them, explaining the purpose of the research, seeing if they will cooperate by searching out earlier letters, if any exist, and providing counseling if they need it. Despite, Lester's objection to this research, this chapter will review the research

---

33 For each suicide note, an individual matched for age and occupational level was asked to write a suicide note. The sample was restricted to Caucasian, Protestant, native-born males aged 25 to 60.

published on genuine versus simulated suicide notes and present the results of an LIWC analysis.

11.1 Guessing which Notes are Genuine

Can the genuine suicide note be distinguished from a simulated note? Osgood and Walker (1959) looked at the matched pairs of genuine and simulated notes published by Shneidman and Farberow. Osgood and Walker had graduate students with no prior experience of suicide notes predict which of each pair was the genuine note. The students performed at exactly the chance level, identifying a mean of 16.5 notes of the 33 pairs correctly. Osgood and Walker themselves carried out the task after reading and comparing a different sample of genuine suicide notes with a sample of ordinary letters. They were correct on 28.5 of the pairs. Therefore, experience with suicide notes increased the accuracy of assignment.

Lester (1993) obtained two sets of genuine and simulated suicide notes (one set from Shneidman and Farberow [1957b] and another set from Seiden and Tauber [1970]) and found that naive judges showed no parallel-forms reliability. He found that expert suicidologists could guess the genuine notes better than chance, while naive judges could not. Lester (1991a) had naive judges guess the genuine note in Shneidman and Farberow's sample of genuine and simulated note pairs, and the odd-even correlation was moderate, suggesting that the judges were reasonably consistent.

Lester (1991b) found the accuracy of naive judges of Shneidman and Farberow's sample of notes was associated with their extraversion scores, but not with their neuroticism or psychoticism scores or with their Keirsey-Bates temperament scores. Lester (1995a) found that Machiavellian scores did not predict the success of naive judges, while Lester (1994c) found that judges more sympathetic to suicide were more accurate in picking out the genuine notes, both studies again using Shneidman and Farberow's sample of notes.

Leenaars and Lester (1991) found that the genuine note in 19 of 33 pairs of genuine and simulated suicide notes was obvious to the student judges, while in 14 of the pairs it was not. Asking the judges for their reasons for judging a note to be genuine, it appeared that the students looked for traumatic events and idiosyncratic views to judge a suicide note to be genuine.

11.2 Differences between Genuine and Simulated Suicide Notes

Shneidman and Farberow (1957a) compared their genuine and simulated notes for the quality of the thought units in them using a coding system devised by Dollard and Mowrer (1947). The genuine notes had significantly more statements overall than the simulated notes, but did not differ in the proportion of discomfort statements (discomfort statements divided by the sum of relief plus discomfort statements).[34] They noted informally that the type of discomfort statements differed in the genuine and simulated notes. The genuine notes had deeper feelings of hatred, vengeance and self-blame. However, this difference was not tested in a quantitative way by the authors. Shneidman and Farberow commented that the excess of neutral statements in the genuine notes possibly reflected a tendency on the part of the suicidal person to confuse the self as experienced by the self with the self as experienced by others, but I do not follow their reasoning here.

Spiegel and Neuringer (1963) argued that an individual does not necessarily complete suicide when the urge to die becomes stronger than the urge to live. What is necessary is that the dread that rises as the individual approaches a suicidal action needs to be reduced in some way. Spiegel and Neuringer argued that the defenses that are used to reduce dread might include self-deception over the imminent suicidal action, a tendency to avoid mention of suicide, and a tendency to concentrate on topics other than suicide. Psychotic processes, which would serve to protect the individual from realizing the implications of the suicidal action, might be reflected in the disorganization of the note.

These defenses were operationally measured by the following five attributes: relative explicitness of expressed suicidal intention, dramatic quality of the note, disorganization of thought processes, presence of the word "suicide" or suicide synonyms, and presence of instructions to the reader with respect to the disposal of property or the assumption of responsibilities. The results confirmed four of the five hypotheses: the genuine notes had less explicitness, fewer mentions of suicide, a greater number of instructions, and greater disorganization. There was no difference in dramatic quality.

Osgood and Walker (1959) argued that the suicidal individual has a heightened drive level, and they hypothesized that this would lead to greater stereotypy and greater disorganization in suicide notes than in ordinary letters. Since drive states are characterized by distinctive cues which have a directive function, they hypothesized that suicide notes should be characterized by increased frequency of those grammatical and lexical choices associated with motives leading to self-destruction. Finally, if several motives are operating, suicide notes should show greater evidence of conflict. To test these hypotheses, they compared a sample of suicide notes and a sample of ordinary letters written by nonsuicidal people matched for sex and age.

The suicide notes were more stereotyped than the letters: they had a smaller proportion of different words used, they had more repetition of phrases, there were fewer adjectival and adverbial qualifiers (as compared to the number of nouns and verbs), and they had more definitive terms (like always and never). The suicide notes of men were more redundant than the letters, but the difference for women was not

34 The statistical analysis presented in Shneidman and Farberow's paper appears to be incorrect.

significant. There were no significant differences in the average number of syllables per word.[35]

There were no differences between the suicide notes and the letters in disorganization–there were no differences in syntactical, grammar, spelling or punctuation errors. For women, there were no differences in the sentence length but, for men, the suicides notes had longer sentences, contrary to the prediction of Osgood and Walker who thought that, under stress, sentence length would decrease.

There was evidence of a directive state–the suicide notes had a higher proportion of discomfort statements, more evaluative common-meaning terms (like unfair and sweetheart), fewer positive evaluative assertions (a measure that is correlated with the proportion of discomfort statements), and more mands (utterances such as imperatives, which express a need of the speaker and require some reaction from the reader for their satisfaction). There was no difference in the distribution of past, present, and future references, whereas Osgood and Walker had predicted more emphasis on the past in suicide, notes. There was evidence for a state of conflict–the suicide notes had verbs with more qualifications (for example, "used to be good" rather than "was good"), more ambivalent constructions (such as but, should, maybe, and except), and more ambivalent evaluative assertions.

Osgood and Walker then applied their findings to Shneidman and Farberow's 33 pairs of genuine and simulated suicide notes. Only 13 pairs of notes had sufficient length for a meaningful analysis. For stereotypy, only the measure of adjective-adverb/noun-verb ratio significantly differentiated the genuine from the simulated notes. (The redundancy measure was not used since the notes were too brief.) The mand measure of the directive state differentiated the two groups and, although the ambivalent construction measure of conflict differentiated the groups, the direction was opposite to that in the first part of the study. Disorganization measures were not investigated since they had not been found to be of use in the first part of the study. Eliminating those measures which failed to differentiate suicide notes from letters (structural disturbances, average length of sentences, and time orientation), those measures susceptible to faking (the proportion of discomfort statements, evaluative terms, and positive evaluative assertions), and the redundancy measure (since the notes were too brief for a meaningful application), Osgood and Walker applied the remaining nine measures to predict which of the notes in the 13 pairs were the genuine ones. The predictions were correct for 10 pairs, a significant difference.

To investigate further the stereotypy of the genuine notes, Osgood and Walker catalogued the words used by more than five of the writers of each group of notes. The genuine writers used more words in common than did the nonsuicidal writers. A content analysis showed that the genuine suicide notes had more terms of endearment

35 Osgood and Walker had argued that shorter words tend to be more frequent than longer words (Zipf, 1949) and so should indicated stereotypy.

and references to mother, whereas the simulated notes contained more abstractions and references to insurance. Genuine notes had more verbs of simple action (go, tell) whereas simulated notes had more verbs referring to mental states (know, think). The genuine notes had more references to positive states (such as love and hope).

Osgood and Walker noted that possibly other models could have predicted their results. However, they felt that an explanation based on differences in educational and intelligence levels of the two groups of writers was unlikely to be valid since there were no differences in disorganization between the suicide notes and letters.

Tuckman and Ziegler (1966) examined the 33 pairs of genuine and simulated notes for differences in social maturity. They measured social maturity using the ontogenetic sequence observed by Piaget (1926) in the speech of children, in which the child moves away from the use of self terms (I, me) toward self-other terms (we, us) and finally to other terms (you, them). They predicted that the genuine notes should have a greater emphasis on self-reference than on other-reference. To test this, they counted the number of different categories of pronouns in the notes. The notes did not differ in the total number of different categories of pronouns or in the proportions. Tuckman and Ziegler concluded that the simulated notes may have been written in a state of anxiety and that this may have led to as low a level of social maturity as shown by the suicidal individuals.

Another study of content was carried out by Gottschalk and Gleser (1960) who had no hypotheses. They coded the words used in the 33 pairs of genuine and simulated notes into grammatical categories and psychological categories. The genuine notes had fewer prepositions, fewer conjunctions and more substantives than the simulated notes. There were no differences in the proportions of adjectives, adverbs, interjections, verbs, or total number of words. With regard to psychological categories, there were fewer words denoting reflective or cognitive process in the genuine notes. There were no differences in the proportion of words denoting feeling or motivation, perceptual processes, activity or movement, relationships in time or space, measures of quantity, or negation. Finally, there were no differences with regard to references to the self, animals or flowers, or to the person addressed. The genuine notes did have more references to others and to objects.

One complexity introduced by the authors in this study was that they analyzed the results in two ways: treating the notes as matched pairs and as independent groups. The results reported above were for matched-pairs analyses. The results of the analysis for independent groups differed. The only common significant differences were for substantives, references to others, and references to objects.

Gottschalk and Gleser then obtained a new sample of genuine suicide notes. For the signs that they had had identified in the first part of the study, no differences were found in the new sample for men as compared to women or for married people as compared to single people. When the new sample was compared to the simulated notes of the first part of the study, the results of the first part were replicated. Gottschalk and Gleser felt that the differences that they reported reflected the nature of the genuine suicide note as a communication to another, but they did not explain their reasoning here.

Ogilvie, et al. (1965) compared the same 33 pairs of genuine and simulated notes using a computer program to carry out a content analysis. The genuine notes had more references to "things" such as roles and objects. The simulated notes had more references to emotional states and actions. For the sentences containing a reference to the female role, it was found that the genuine note writes gave fewer instructions to females, gave more information about females, and made more references to being acted upon by a female than did the simulated note writers.[36] Looking at the instructions given to females, the genuine note writers gave more specific instructions and fewer vague instructions.

Looking at actions, Ogilvie, et al. found that the genuine writers used the concept of "think" in the context of knowing or decision making ("I think that if I went to the doctor, I would. . .), whereas the simulated note writers used the concept more in attempting to solve a problem ("I am thinking of all the problems we have shared"). Ogilvie, et al. noted the similarity of their results to those of Gottschalk and Gleser discussed above. Since the two sets of workers were using the same data and similar analyses, this is not surprising. Using three items (reference to concrete things, places and persons, use of the word love in the text, and total number of references to processes of thought and decision), the authors were able to classify 30 of the 33 pairs of notes correctly.

Henken (1976) used a computer program to compare the genuine suicide notes, simulated suicide notes and notes written by people about to die. The genuine notes were more concrete, constricted and concerned with interpersonal relationships (especially those with the opposite sex). Edelman and Renshaw (1982) also compared the genuine and simulated notes by computer analysis and found the genuine notes to be longer with fewer positive modifiers. The genuine notes had more negatives (e.g., "not"), authority (e.g., proper nouns), audience (e.g., "you") and generalized others (e.g., third-person pronouns), modified nouns, modified verbs, cognizance of objects (concrete objects), modification of objects and actions, negative modification, negative modification of known people and positive modification of unknown people, and static action, and fewer references to future time.

Lester (1971b) found no difference between Shneidman and Farberow's genuine and simulated suicide notes in the need for affiliation expressed in them. Lester (1973) found no differences in the tense of the verbs in the notes, although the genuine notes did have more verbs in the conditional tense and more imperatives. Lester (1989c) found that the genuine notes more often had content reflecting the desire to kill (anger) but did not differ in the desires to be killed (depression and guilt) and to die (escape).

---

36 Remember, all of the note writers were male.

Lester and Leenaars (1988) found that the genuine notes contained more direct accusations and wills/testaments and fewer conventional "first-form" notes (i.e., notes that focus on conventional explanations and pleas for forgiveness). McLister and Leenaars (1988; Leenaars, et al., 1989) found more signs of unconscious forces at play in the genuine notes than in the simulated notes (as well as more mention of spouses and fathers). Black (1993) found that the genuine notes were longer and, after controls for length, had more instructions, information, religious ideas and dates. The simulated notes had more depression, justification, life seen as overwhelming as a reason for suicide, and less mention of the after-life.

11.3 Testing Alfred Adler's Theory of Suicide

Darbonne (1967) compared a different sample of suicide notes written by a group of white American men who had completed suicide with simulated notes written by men matched for race, age, and occupation and simluated notes by white American men who were currently threatening suicide. The hypotheses tested by Darbonne derived from Adler's views on suicide (Ansbacher, 1961).

Adler maintained that the suicidal individual was characterized by a pampered life style and dependency. The notes of completed suicides as compared to the simulated notes more often mentioned a need to have things done for them, a heightened concern with whether or not they had received emotional support from others, and the importance of parental figures to them. There were no significant differences in the difficulties experienced in adapting to loss.

There was less support for the notion that the completed suicides would be characterized by inferiority feelings and self-centered goals. There were no differences between the two sets of notes in direct expressions of low self-esteem or self-praise, feelings of being at the mercy of external forces, or in the number of self-referents. However, there were more references by the completed suicides to other people than there were by the nonsuicidal persons, and there were also more mentions of the absence or breaking of social ties. Darbonne felt that these last two comparisons were relevant to feelings of inferiority and self-centered goals, but they seem to me to be more relevant to the dependency of the person.

Adler hypothesized that suicides would be very active, and Darbonne found that the completed suicides used more verbs referring to physical motor behavior than did the nonsuicidal persons, and their notes contained more verbs and adjectives. However, the notes did not differ in length (a measure of verbal activity), and there was no difference by the method of suicide used or chosen by the subject. (The methods of suicide had been previously rated by psychologists for the degree of activity involved.)

There was some support for the notion that the notes from completed suicides would show more veiled aggression than the simluated notes. The notes of the completed suicides had more veiled hostility, more frequent mentions of concern regarding the blame of others for their suicide, and more concern with informing others and addressing the note to others as compared to the simulated notes. However, the two sets of notes did not differ in expressions of direct anger, mentions of suffering, and feelings that others had been hurt by the past behavior of the note writer.

Overall, the results supported Darbonne's predictions based upon Adlerian ideas about suicide, with the exception of the hypothesized differences in inferiority feelings. Each idea tested by Darbonne received some support, and none of the tests produced significant results in a direction opposite to that predicted. The eleven variables that had proved successful in differentiating the notes of the completed suicides from those of the nonsuicidal persons were used to compare the notes of those threatening suicide with those of the two other groups. With regard to veiled aggression and a pampered life style and dependency, those threatening suicide resembled the completed suicides in inferiority feelings and self-centered goals but resembled the nonsuicidal persons in activity. Those threatening suicide were divided into a high risk and a low risk group. The two groups did not differ on any of the eleven variables significantly. The resemblance of those threatening suicide with the completed suicides perhaps reflects the degree to which those threatening suicide possess high suicidal potential. However, the comparison of the high and low risk group among those threatening suicide failed to reveal differences, and so interpretation of the results from those threatening suicide is not easy.

11.4 Testing Other Theories of Suicide

Leenaars formulated several theories of suicide into specific statements and examined the presence of these statements in Shneidman and Farberow's 33 pairs of genuine and simulated suicide notes. Leenaars (1988a) found that genuine notes contained more of the themes based on the theories of Sigmund Freud, Edwin Shneidman, and Gregory Zilboorg, and to a lesser extent Henry Murray and Harry Sullivan, but not from the theories of Alfred Adler, Ludwig Binswanger, Carl Jung, or George Kelly. Balance and Leenaars (1986) found that the genuine and simulated notes had different frequencies for statements derived from Aaron Beck's theory of suicide. The genuine notes had more magnification, minimization and overgeneralization, while the simulated notes had more hopelessness, suffering and desire for escape. Lester and Leenaars (1987) compared the genuine notes of each pair which naïve subjects could easily identify correctly with those which were hard to identify. The protocol sentences used by Leenaars in his research failed to differentiate these two sets of genuine notes.

11.5 Handwriting

Frederick (1968) investigated whether suicide notes could be distinguished using handwriting. He had a sample of genuine notes typed and had handwritten copies made from the typed copies by individuals matched with the suicidal writers for sex and age. The paper used for the note was matched with the original note for size, color, type of paper, and amount of wear. Frederick used three sets of judges. Graphologists identified the genuine notes at a level better than chance, while detectives and secretaries both performed at chance level. There was no apparent effect on the accuracy of the judgments from the type of paper used for the note or from the sex and age of the writers.

11.6 The LIWC Analysis

The 33 pairs of genuine and simulated suicide notes from the book written by Shneidman and Farberow (1957b) were run through the LIWC. All were from Caucasian, Protestant, native-born men ages 25-59 years. Shneidman and Farberow matched the writers of these genuine and simulated for age and occupation, and so the scores can be treated as paired data.

Paired t-tests identified 10 significant differences out of 76 (see Table 11.1). The genuine notes were longer and had fewer words per sentence, fewer unique words, more pronouns, more second person pronouns such as "you," fewer prepositions, more numbers, fewer words related to causation such as "because" and "hence," more words concerned with social processes such as "talk" and "friend," and more references to people. It appears, therefore, that the genuine notes were more concerned with other people and less focused on explaining why the individual is choosing to die by suicide. Interestingly, there were no differences in content categories, including school or work, leisure activities, religion, death and dying, body states and symptoms, or sex and sexuality.[37]

These results did not confirm the differences reported by Osgood and Walker (1959) reviewed above in positive emotions or optimism, but the results did confirm that the genuine notes had fewer references to cognitive processes and causation. Unlike the results reported by Tuckman and Ziegler (1966) who found no differences in pronouns, the present analysis found more references to "you" in the genuine notes. However, Gottschalk and Gleser's (1960) results concerning pronouns did match the present results.

37 Treating the data as two independent samples and using point-biserial correlation coefficients, the same 10 significant differences were identified as those found in the paired-sample analysis.

Tab. 11.1: Differences between simulated and genuine notes (mean scores shown)

	Genuine notes	Simulated notes
Word count	108.88	65.67*
Words per sentence	10.90	14.35*
Unique words	71.24	80.12*
Pronouns	20.62	16.68*
Total second person	5.43	3.38*
Prepositions	9.16	11.65*
Numbers	1.08	0.28*
Causation	0.50	1.53*
Social processes	12.37	8.71**
Other references to people	7.81	5.27*

* two-tailed p < .05, ** two-tailed p < .01

11.7 A Second Sample of Simulated Suicide Notes

Seiden and Tauber (1970) also collected a sample of genuine and simulated suicide notes, and these notes were also analyzed by the LIWC program (see Table 11.2). There were 17 significant differences. The genuine suicide notes had shorter sentences, fewer dictionary words, less use of "we," fewer articles and prepositions, more use of numbers, more affect (emotion) and especially positive emotions, less use of cognitive mechanisms, including causation and discrepancies, more tentative words, more references to seeing, more references to family, and more words concerned with "down" and "exclusion."

Which differences were similar in this set of genuine and simulated suicide notes and those from Shneidman and Farberow? In both sets, the genuine notes had shorter sentences, fewer prepositions and more numbers, and less concern with causation. It appears, then, that simulated note writers try to explain the reasons for their suicide more than the genuine notes writers and write longer sentences in order to do this. The greater use of numbers in the genuine suicide notes may reflect the greater amount of instructions and directions (such as whom to contact and to whom various objects and money is to be given). The numbers were most likely telephone numbers and street addresses.

11.8 Pseudocides

Seiden and Tauber (1970) also collected a sample of notes left by people who had possibly pretended to kill themselves from the Golden Gate Bridge. These cases had no eye-witness to the jump and no body was found. From 134 possible cases, 34 appeared to be "suspicious," and 24 of these were established as "definite." Ten of these were

Tab. 11.2: A comparison of genuine, simulated and hoax suicide notes (point biserial correlation shown)

	Genuine v. Simulated notes	**Hoax v. simulated notes**	**Hoax v. genuine notes**
Word count	-0.22	0.28#	0.37*
Words per sentence	-0.53**	-0.52**	0.04
Unique words	0.29#	-0.10	-0.32*
Words in the dictionary	-0.50**	-0.33*	0.29#
Words longer than 6 letters	-0.04	-0.37*	-0.25
First person plural	-0.32*	-0.30#	0.20
Total third person	-0.15	0.17	0.38*
Articles	-0.48**	-0.05	0.39**
Prepositions	-0.54**	-0.34*	0.22
Numbers	0.33*	0.31*	-0.22
Affect	0.33*	0.23	-0.18
Positive emotions	0.37*	0.14	-0.27#
Positive feelings	0.29#	0.15	-0.14
Cognitive processes	-0.56**	-0.34*	0.34*
Causation	-0.35*	-0.29#	0.13
Insight	-0.30#	-0.34*	0.05
Discrepancies	-0.46**	-0.01	0.43**
Tentative	-0.36*	-0.20	0.20
Seeing	-0.31*	-0.09	0.25
Family	0.31*	0.01	-0.31*
Future tense verbs	-0.27#	0.01	0.26
Down	-0.31*	-0.08	0.38**
Exclusive	-0.48**	-0.08	0.38*
School	0.16	0.36*	0.26
Religion	0.28#	0.18	-0.21
Death	-0.11	-0.37*	-0.13
Eating	-	0.28#	0.28#
Sexual	0.30#	0.19	-0.12

* two-tailed p < .05, ** two-tailed p < .01, # trends (two-tailed p < .10)

later arrested for crimes other than being a missing person. These pseudocides showed little depression prior to their action or social withdrawal. They tended to be impulsive individuals who acted-out non-violently.

Seiden and Tauber reported that the pseudocide notes from 21 individuals were longer than the genuine and simulated notes, although with a much greater variability in length. The pseudocide notes gave more realistic reasons for their suicide (such as mentioning financial and legal problems more), contained more emotion, and were more explicit about their suicide as compared to the genuine notes. Lester, et al. (1990) found that anger (Menninger's "to kill" motive) was present more often in the pseudocide notes than in the genuine or simulated notes, while self-blame (Menninger's "to be killed" motive) was present more often in the genuine suicide notes and the desire to escape less often present.

The 21 pseudocide notes were compared, using the LIWC program with the 21 genuine and the 21 simulated notes from the same study, and the results are shown in Table 11.2. The pseudocide and simulated notes differed significantly on ten variables, while the pseudocide and genuine notes differed significantly on nine variables. Thus, the pseudocide notes did not resemble the genuine suicide notes either more or less than they resembled the simulated suicide notes. They appear to constitute a third type of note, different in many respects from both genuine and simulated suicide notes.

This makes sense since the writers of pseudocide notes are, presumably, not suicidal, and so their notes should differ from genuine suicide notes. On the other hand, they are probably in the midst of a major crisis and feeling desperate since they are faking their own suicide and starting a new life with a different identity. Thus, their notes should differ from simulated suicide notes which are typically written by people who are neither suicidal nor in a major crisis.

12 Suicide Notes From Attempted and Completed Suicides

An interesting question is whether the suicide notes written by those attempt suicide resemble or differ from the suicide notes written by completed suicides. However, it is not easy to collect suicide notes from attempted suicides since there is typically no police investigation (since, in the United States, no crime has been committed), and any suicide notes that were written are usually destroyed by the attempters or by their significant others.

A sample of suicide notes from attempted suicides was collected by Livermore (1985). She compared suicide notes from 20 completed suicides with those from 20 attempted suicides from one town in America. The suicide notes of completed suicides were more often addressed to someone, contained information about whom to contact, said sorry/forgive me, said I love you/darling, and mentioned depression and financial problems. The completed suicides also more often left multiple notes. The groups did not differ in their use of "first-form" notes (Jacobs, 1967) which focus on conventional explanations and pleas for forgiveness.

Brevard[38] and Lester (1991) found that the completers more often addressed their note to someone, said "sorry," and mentioned grandparents. The notes from the completed suicides had a lower total isolation score obtained by summing these characteristics. The attempters' notes were more often in the nature of a last will and testament. Brevard, et al. (1990) compared these two sets of notes and found that the notes from attempters less often expressed the wish to be killed (anger-in) but did not differ in the wishes to die (escape) or to kill (anger-out). Lester (1994a) confirmed this result after controlling for the sex and age of the note writers. Leenaars, et al. (1992b) matched the notes from the attempted suicides (adding some other notes from attempted suicides in Leenaars's collection of notes) and matched them for age and sex with suicide notes from completed suicides in his collection. They found no differences in Menninger's three motives for suicide (to die, to kill and to be killed) when the notes were matched for age and sex.

Black and Lester (2001), using codings made by raters, found two significant differences out of 52 examined. The notes from completed suicides gave more information and more often asked for forgiveness. However, controls for sex and age eliminated these two differences. Leenaars, et al. (1992a) found no differences in eight suicidal patterns[39] between these notes from attempters and completers. On twenty

---

38 Formerly Livermore.

39 Unbearable psychological pain, interpersonal relations, rejection-aggression, inability to adjust, indirect expressions, identification-egression, ego, and cognitive constriction.

content dimensions, the attempters more often indicated that suicide was a style of life and they seemed to be less well social integrated.

Incidentally, Lester (1994b) found that suicidologists could not distinguish the suicide notes from completers and attempters at a level better than chance, while Black and Lester (1995) found that skilled judges of suicide notes also could not distinguish them from each other at a level better than chance.

The general conclusion from these studies is that the suicide notes from completed suicides indicate more social isolation.

12.1 Tests of Theories of Suicide

Joiner (2005) proposed that a sense of burdensomeness to others (close relatives in particular) is a critical factor in motivating people to choose suicide, a view which is consistent with an evolutionary-psychological (or sociobiological) theory of suicide (De Catanzaro, 1980). De Catanzaro proposed that suicide advances the welfare of the gene pool by removing the genes of those who are less biologically fit (and less able to reproduce), those in poor psychological and physical health and those whose families would be better off without them. Joiner, et al. (2002) predicted that burdensomeness should be more apparent in the notes of completed suicides than in those of attempted suicides. The two sets of notes did not differ in ratings by judges of hopelessness, emotional pain, efforts to control the writers' negative emotions, or efforts to control other people. However, the notes of the completers did have significantly more content reflecting burdensomeness, even after controls for age and sex.[40]

Rogers, et al. (2007) used this sample of notes from completed and attempted suicides to test Rogers' (2001) existential-constructivist theory of suicide. The content of the notes was rated for relational, somatic, spiritual and psychological motivations. The presence of the four types of motivations were, in order, psychological, relational, spiritual and somatic, and the notes from the completed suicides had more relational content than the notes from attempters.

Zhang and Lester (2008) tested a strain theory of suicide (Zhang, 2005) which proposes that four sources of strain characterize suicides: (i) strains from conflicting values, (ii) discrepancies between aspirations and reality, (iii) relative deprivations such as poverty, and (iv) deficient coping skills in the face of crises. The strains were rated as present in the following order of frequency: aspiration, coping, value and deprivation strains. The two sets of notes differed significantly on only one strain–the

---

40 Joiner, et al. also found that, among a sample of notes from German completed suicides, the notes from suicides using more lethal methods for suicide (such as guns and hanging) had more content reflecting burdensomeness than notes from suicides using less lethal methods for suicide (such as medications).

notes from completed suicides had significantly less content reflecting deprivation strains than the notes from attempted suicides.

12.2 The LIWC Analysis

These forty suicide notes were analyzed using the LIWC program.[41] The point-biserial correlations between the outcome of the suicidal act and the LIWC variables are shown in Table 12-1.[42]

Tab. 12.1: Point biserial associations with suicide outcome

	Correlation coefficient
Unique words	-0.31*
Hearing	0.44**
Future tense verbs	0.43**
Total second person	0.30#
Positive emotions	0.30#
Social processes	0.29#
Other references to people	0.31#
Time	-0.30#
Inclusive	-0.31#
School	0.28#
Metaphysical issues	-0.29#
Religion	-0.30#

* two-tailed p < .05, ** two-tailed p < .01, # trend (two-tailed p < 0.10)

The notes from completed suicides more often had content related to references to others ('you'), positive emotions, hearing, social, people in general, future tense and school, and fewer references related to time, inclusive, metaphysics and religion and fewer unique words. The reduced content for "inclusive" involved words such as "with" or "include" might indicate greater social isolation and lack of belongingness in the completed suicides, consistent with Durkheim's (1897) concept of a lack of social integration which he felt characterized suicides and Joiner's (2005) proposal that thwarted belongingness is a necessary precursor to suicide. The notes from completed suicides also had fewer metaphysical references which may be indicative

41 The two sets of suicide notes did not differ in sex or age.

42 Handelman and Lester (2007) carried out a similar LIWC analysis, using two-way ANOVAs (outcome by sex) with similar results.

of "cognitive deconstruction" as described in Baumeister's (1990) escape theory of suicide in which the suicidal individual is conceptualized as endeavoring to escape from their *self.*

Thus, the suicide notes from the attempted suicides indicated greater distress. Their notes had fewer positive emotions, fewer social references, fewer future tense verbs and more metaphysical references. These differences suggest that the attempters were in greater psychological pain *at the time of writing the note,* and more concerned with their own present condition and less concerned with others. The difference is consistent with the improvement in mood noted in completed suicides in the day prior to their death, which has been noted earlier in this book.

12.3 Comment

The findings from this single set of notes from completed and attempted suicides have identified several interesting differences and proved useful for testing emerging theories of suicide. It is important that additional samples of notes from attempted suicides be collected so that the reliability of these findings can be examined.

13 Differences by Gender, Age and Other Variables

The present chapter explores differences in the content of genuine suicide notes by gender, age, marital status and the method chosen for suicide.

13.1 The Suicide Notes of Men and Women

There are strong and clear sex differences in suicidal behavior. Women attempt suicide more than do men, whereas men complete suicide more than do women (Canetto & Lester, 1995). Women use different methods for suicide than do men, preferring medications more and hanging and firearms less (Lester, 1984). It is thought, perhaps erroneously, that the motives behind the suicidal act differ, with women choosing suicide over love crises and men for achievement-oriented crises (Canetto, 1992-1993).

Despite these differences, studies of the suicide notes left by women and men have identified few differences. In an extensive study, Leenaars (1988b) found no differences in content, as have many other studies (Lester, 1989; Lester & Hummel, 1980; Lester & Heim, 1992; Lester & Linn, 1997; Linn & Lester, 1996). In contrast, Black (1989) found more indications of depression, self-hostility, confusion and despondency over the death of others in the suicide notes of women, while Lester and Reeve (1982) found that notes from women had fewer negative emotions but were more disorganized. All of these studies used judges to rate the suicide notes, a technique which can introduce subjectivity and unreliability in the judgments. The present chapter applies the objectivity proved by the LIWC to the analysis of suicide notes.

13.1.1 Samples

(1) Forty suicide notes from completed suicides from a town in Germany. There were 20 men and 20 women whose mean age was 35.5 years (*SD* = 18.8). The men and women did not differ in age.
(2) Forty-eight suicide notes from completed suicides from a town in the United States. There were 34 men and 14 women whose mean age was 43.2 years (*SD* = 17.5). The men and women did not differ in age.
(3) Two hundred and sixty one suicide notes from completed suicides in Tasmania, Australia: There were 195 men and 65 women with one subject with missing data. Their mean age was 41.8 yrs. (*SD* = 17.1). The men and women did not differ in age.

13.1.2 Results

The results are shown in Table 13-1.

Tab. 13.1: Sex differences in the content of suicide notes

	Germany n=40	America n=48	Australia n=260
Word count	0.44**	-0.22	0.01
Unique words	-0.49***	0.17	-0.03
Words in dictionary	0.10	0.29*	-0.15*
Pronouns	0.06	0.13	-0.17**
First person singular	-0.22	0.11	-0.16**
First person plural	0.18	0.08	-0.16**
Total first person	-0.20	0.12	-0.18**
Negation	-0.48**	-0.07	-0.17**
Articles	0.22	0.12	0.18**
Numbers	0.10	-0.28*	0.14*
Positive feelings	-0.02	0.17	-0.13*
Cognit9ve processes	-0.39*	0.14	-0.14*
Insight	-0.31#	0.04	-0.15*
Discrepancies	-0.28	0.03	-0.16*
Tentative	-0.35*	-0.01	-0.05
Senses	0.04	-0.28#	0.04
Hearing	0.10	-0.29*	-0.01
Other refs to people	0.30#	0.01	-0.09
Friends	0.30#	-0.27#	0.04
Time	0.27#	0.05	-0.01
Present tense verbs	0.08	0.04	-0.23***
Up	-0.27#	-0.13	0.01
Down	0.32*	-0.09	0.09
Inclusive	0.27#	0.09	-0.01
Money	0.29#	0.20	0.04
Sleep	0.22	-0.26#	-0.10#

* two-tailed p < .05, ** two-tailed p < .01, *** two-tailed p < .001, # trend (two-tailed p < 0.10)

13.1.2.1 German Sample

Seven significant associations were found: men wrote longer notes, with fewer unique words, fewer negations, less mention of cognitive mechanism (such as cause, know, ought), fewer insight words (such as think, know, consider), fewer tentative words (such as maybe, perhaps), and more words concerned with "down" (such as down, below, under). Another eight associations showed trends: the men used few discrepancy words (such as should, would, could), communication words (such as talk, share, converse) and words concerned with "up", but had more references to people, friends, time, inclusion (such as with, and, include), and money.

Overall, the notes of men were more concerned with mentions of others, including friends, and less concerned with causation, and so the notes of the men seemed to be less concerned with explaining the reasons for their suicide and more concerned with communicating with others.

13.1.2.2 American Sample

Only three significant differences were found, no more than would be expected on the basis of chance with so many variables. The women used numbers more, words related to hearing more, and fewer dictionary words. These differences have little psychological significance.

13.1.2.3 Australian Sample

Thirteen significant differences were found between the content of the notes from men and women. The notes from women had a higher percentage of words found in the dictionary, pronouns, "I," "we," references to the self, negations, positive feelings, references to cognitive processes, insight words, discrepancy words (such as should, would and could), and present tense verbs, and a lower percentage of articles (such as a, an, the), and numbers.

13.1.3 Comment

The results of the study of German suicide notes differed greatly from those of American suicide notes, indicating perhaps a lack of generality in the results. These two samples were small, and so the results from the much larger Australian sample may be more meaningful. In this Australian sample, women were more concerned with themselves and others and with reasons for their suicide, similar to the results from the German suicide notes. It may be that the notes from men contained more instructions and were less personal. At least two of the three samples agreed for the categories of negations, cognitive mechanisms and insight, and sleep, with men having less of this content than did the women. Since previous research had identified few differences between the suicide notes from men and women, the present analysis provides hypotheses for future research, which clearly need to be tested using large samples.

13.2 Differences across the Life Span

Leenaars (1989) reviewed research on differences in the psychodynamics of suicide by age and the extent to which these differences are reflected in the suicide notes that people write. The suicides of young people are more often motivated by interpersonal conflicts while the suicides of the elderly are more often motivated by internal events, in particular depression and medical illnesses. The suicide notes of younger people more often have inward-directed anger, and the content is more harsh and self-critical. Leenaars's own study found more inward-directed aggression, unsatisfied needs, self-punishment and interpersonal conflicts in the notes of younger adults (aged 18-25) as compared to older adults (aged 55-77).

To examine differences by age, the same samples as those used above were used.

13.2.1 Results

13.2.1.1 German Sample

Only four significant associations were found for age (see Table 13-2): older people used more prepositions, more words concerned with communication, more future tense verbs, and more words concerned with space.

13.2.1.2 American Sample

Only three significant differences were found for age (see Table 13-2): older people used more long words (more than 6 letters) and religious words, and a smaller proportion of words concerned with negative emotions.

13.2.1.3 Australian Sample

Twenty-four significant differences in the content of the notes were found by age (see Table 13-2). The notes of older note writers had fewer words, fewer words per sentence, a lower percentage of words found in the dictionary, pronouns, "I," references to the self, "you," articles, positive feelings, anxiety or fear, references to cognitive processes, causation, tentative words (such as maybe and perhaps), seeing, social processes, references to people, references to family, present tense verbs, exclusive words (such as but and except), sports, and sex and sexuality, and a higher percentage of references to the body and unique words.

13.2.2 Discussion

Clearly, having a larger sample (from Australia) increased the chances of finding significant associations. The major differences in the Australian sample were that the older suicides were less concerned with emotions (positive and negative), with explanations for their suicide, and with social relationships. They did mention the body more, most likely concerning illness and pain (although these categories are not assessed

Tab. 13.2: Correlations over age

	Germany n=40	America[43] n=45	Australia n=258
Word count	-0.14	0.02	-0.13*
Words per sentence	0.15	-0.23	-0.21***
Unique words	0.11	0.10	0.21***
Words in dictionary	-0.04	-0.16	-0.17**
Words with 6+ letters	0.15	0.47***	0.07
Pronouns	-0.22	0.04	-0.29***
First person singular	-0.20	0.01	-0.24***
Total first person	-0.17	0.01	-0.25***
Total second person	-0.02	0.05	-0.16*
Total third person	-0.02	-0.24	-0.12#
Articles	0.23	-0.07	-0.17**
Prepositions	0.40*	0.03	0.11#
Positive feelings	0.18	0.07	-0.16*
Negative emotions	0.03	-0.33*	0.02
Anxiety	-0.07	0.09	-0.14*
Anger	-0.29#	-0.23	0.01
Cognitive processes	-0.21	-0.11	-0.25***
Causation	-0.09	0.01	-0.24***
Insight	-0.08	0.03	-0.12#
Discrepancies	-0.08	0.06	-0.27***
Inhibition	-0.25	-0.26#	0.02
Tentative	-0.03	0.13	-0.16*
Seeing	0.15	-0.02	-0.12#
Social processes	0.10	0.05	-0.21***

43 Three suicides had missing data for age.

continued Tab. 13.2: Correlations over age

	Germany n=40	America[43] n=45	Australia n=258
Communication	0.33*	0.21	-0.07
Other refs to people	0.01	0.01	-0.20**
Family	-0.01	0.16	-0.12*
Past tense verbs	-0.25	-0.28#	-0.07
Present tense verbs	-0.25	0.01	-0.17**
Future tense verbs	0.38*	0.06	-0.08
Space	0.42**	0.16	0.03
Up	0.28#	0.14	0.07
Down	0.18	0.25#	-0.01
Inclusive	0.12	-0.29#	-0.02
Exclusive	-0.21	-0.07	-0.22***
Occupations	-0.05	-0.26#	0.02
Achievements	-0.16	-0.25#	0.06
Sports	0.22	-0.04	-0.13*
Religion	0.27#	0.33*	0.09
Body	0.23	0.14	0.14*
Sexual	-0.13	-0.16	-0.16**
Sleep	0.19	0.20	0.11#
Swearing	-0.29#	0.18	-0.08

* two-tailed p < .05, ** two-tailed p < .01, *** two-tailed p < .001, # trend (two-tailed p < 0.10)

by the LIWC). The notes of the older adults were shorter and probably concerned with instructions (although, again, instructions are not directly assessed by the LIWC).

13.3 Differences by Method of Suicide

Some of the samples of suicide notes analyzed above had data also on the method used for suicide. In the past, research has not identified many psychological differences between those using different methods for suicide. For example, Lester (1971c, 1971d) failed to find differences in the content of suicide notes of those using violent versus non-violent methods for suicide. Lester (1988b) found no differences in the MMPI scores of those using firearms and those using overdoses for suicide. On the other hand, Lester and Beck (1980-1981) found that attempted suicides who used cutting (versus medications) had less suicidal intent, different stressful life events (for example, more often recent legal problems), more severe psychiatric disturbance and more alcohol abuse.

Correlates of choice of method for suicide were explored in these three samples of suicide notes.

13.3.1 Results

13.3.1.1 German Sample

Those using hanging (coded as 1, n = 12) versus solids, liquids or gas (coded as 0, n = 17) used fewer causation words, leisure words, words connected with the home, and words concerned with death (see Table 13-3).

13.3.1.2 American Sample

Comparing those using pills (coded as 1, n = 19) versus firearms (coded as 0, n = 15), those using firearms scored lower on the use of words concerned with discrepancies (such as would, should and could) (see Table 13-3).

Tab. 13.3: Difference in suicide note content by method

	Germany n=29	America n=34
Words per sentence	-0.33#	0.14
Cognitive processes	-0.32#	0.05
Causation	-0.37*	0.29#
Discrepancies	-0.28	-0.46**
Present tense verbs	-0.32#	0.01
Leisure	-0.44*	0.29
Home	-0.38*	0.17
Death	-0.42*	0.08

* two-tailed p < .05, ** two-tailed p < .01, # trend (two-tailed p < 0.10)

13.3.1.3 Australian Sample

In this large sample, three methods were used frequently for suicide: solids and liquids (n=63), guns (n=98) and gas (n=42). These three groups differed on only seven variables (see Table 13-4). Those using guns had a lower percentage of words concerned with sadness/depression and future tense verbs. Those using gas had more references to friends, words concerned with "down," exclusion words (such as but and except), occupation and achievement. Those using solids and liquids had the most references to sadness/depression and future tense verbs.

13.3.2 Discussion

These results are interesting because they suggest that the choice of method for suicide may be related to important psychodynamic characteristics of the individual and, therefore, provide clues to the motives and causes of the suicide. For example, in the Australian sample, depression was more common in those using solids and liquids than in those using guns, suggesting that those using guns may be in an acute crisis (and perhaps acting impulsively), whereas those using solids and liquids may more often have a chronic psychiatric condition. These hypotheses obviously require further research, but they suggest the relevance of choice of method for suicide and possible preventive measures.[44]

Tab. 13.4: Differences by method for the Australian suicide notes- means scores shown

	Solids/liquids	Guns	Gas
Articles*	2.9	3.7	4.2
Future tense verbs*	2.3	1.4	2.1
Down*	0.1	0.1	0.5
Exclusive**	1.9	2.3	3.3
Occupations*	0.7	0.8	1.5
Achievements*	0.4	0.5	1.1
Sad#	0.51	0.26	0.38
Friends#	0.10	0.10	0.60

* two-tailed p < .05, ** two-tailed p < .01, # trend (two-tailed p < 0.10)

44 For a comparison of those using different methods for suicide in this Australian sample on demographic and other personal variables, see Haines, Williams and Lester (2010).

13.4 Marital Status

Hitherto, there has been no research on differences in the content of suicide notes by marital status. Do single, married, divorced and widowed suicides write different suicide notes? This question was explored in these samples of suicide notes.

13.4.1 Results

13.4.1.1 German Sample

Comparing the married suicides (coded as 1, n = 19) with the single individuals (coded as 0, n = 14) there were no significant associations with marital status (see Table 13-5). Since marital status was associated with age and sex, partial correlation coefficients were calculated controlling for age and sex, and the results remained pretty much the same.

Tab. 13.5: Differences by marital status

	Germany (n=33)		America (n=32)	
	r	partial r	r	partial r
Pronouns	-0.09	-0.04	0.36*	0.31#
Total third person	-0.28	-0.31	0.01	0.10
Numbers	-0.12	-0.04	-0.32#	-0.30
Negative emotions	-0.17	0.03	-0.35#	-0.30
Sad	0.06	0.01	-0.44*	-0.44*
Senses	0.16	-0.02	-0.38*	-0.34#
Feeling	0.01	0.03	-0.34#	-0.39*
Communication	0.27	0.03	-0.13	-0.23
Present tense verbs	-0.22	0.05	0.30#	0.25
Inclusive	0.23	-0.15	-0.31#	-0.26
Motion	0.15	0.00	0.42*	0.34#
Occupations	0.25	0.12	-0.37*	-0.31
Achievements	0.09	0.19	-0.38*	-0.36#
Leisure	-0.29	-0.28	-0.11	-0.11
Home	-0.25	-0.28	-0.34#	-0.36#
Death	-0.18	-0.47*	-0.31#	-0.33#
Sleep	-0.01	0.24	-0.05	-0.08
Swearing	-0.27	-0.10	0.09	-0.03

* two-tailed $p < .05$, ** two-tailed $p < .01$, # trend (two-tailed $p < 0.10$)

13.4.1.2 American Sample

Comparing the suicide notes from married individuals (coded as 1, n = 19) with those from the single suicides (coded as 0, n = 13), six significant differences were identified (see Table 13-5). The notes from married individuals had more pronouns and references to motion, and fewer references to sadness, the senses, occupation and achievement. Since marital status was associated with both age and sex, partial correlation coefficients were calculated controlling for age and sex, and the results remained similar.

13.4.1.3 Australian Sample

As before, comparing the married and single suicides and the married and divorced suicides revealed many more differences than in the smaller German and American samples (see Table 13-6). The married suicides wrote shorter notes than the never married suicides, had more positive emotions and fewer negative emotions, and were less concerned with explaining their behavior. Compared to the divorced suicides, the married suicides again wrote shorter suicide notes but did not substantially in the emotions expressed. This might be because the married suicides were often in the midst of marital conflict, and so were concerned with similar issues as the divorced suicides. The married suicides were again somewhat less concerned with explaining their behavior.

13.4.2 Discussion

Since this is the first study of the suicides notes of single, married and divorced suicides, it may provide hypotheses for future research. As before, more significant findings were identified with the larger (Australian) sample, emphasizing the importance of sample size in this type of research.

13.4.3 Comments

The analyses in this chapter have identified several interesting hypotheses for future research. Whereas previous research had identified few differences between the suicide notes of men and women, the present analysis of the Australian sample identified a number of interesting differences, such as more positive emotions and references to cognitive processes in the suicide notes of women. Differences were also found by age, marital status and the method chosen for suicide.

Previous research was constrained by the small sample sizes, but the Australian sample of 261 suicides notes demonstrates that obtaining a large sample of suicide notes produces results that are significant and, because of the large sample size, likely to be more reliable results. Future research on suicide notes should make an effort to obtain large sample sizes. Sample sizes of wenty or thirty suicide notes are not enough for meaningful research.

Tab. 13.6: Differences by marital status for the Australian sample

	Married versus Single (coded as 1 versus 0) n = 168		**Married versus Divorced (coded as 1 versus 0) n = 158**	
	Pearson correlations	Partial correlations	Pearson correlations	Partial correlations
Word count	-.21**	-.16*	-.29***	-.30***
Words per sentence	-.22**	-.12	-.18*	-.18*
Unique words	.23**	.16*	.31***	.32***
Total second person	.07	.18*	.03	.05
Total third person	-.07	-.04	-.26***	-.25**
Affect	.16*	.13#	.08	.07
Positive emotions	.20**	.18*	.12	.11
Positive feelings	.19*	.24**	.13	.15#
Anxiety	-.13#	-.07	.09	.05
Sad	-.13#	-.10	-.18*	-.19*
Cognitive processes	-.20*	-.15#	-.09	-.16*
Causation	-.29***	-.21**	-.19*	-.19*
Discrepancies	-.16*	-.10	-.13	-.18*
Social processes	.07	.19*	-.07	-.06
Other refs to people	.07	.16*	-.06	-.05
Humans	.17*	.22**	-.13	-.11
Present tense verbs	.15#	.19*	.17*	.14#
Up	.16*	.14#	.14#	.14#
Inclusive	-.07	-.09	-.11	-.14#
Religion	.15#	.13#	-.02	-.04
Death	-.11	-.13#	-.09	-.09
Physical states	.15#	.16*	.13#	.17*
Sexual	.17*	.22**	.14#	.16#
Eating	.08	.06	.13#	.14#
Grooming	-.12	-.18*	-.07	-.08
Swearing	.07	.13#	-.02	.01

* two-tailed $p < .05$, ** two-tailed $p < .01$, *** two-tailed $p < .001$, # trend (two-tailed $p < .10$)

14 Protest Suicide in Korean Students and Laborers[45]

Protest suicide has a long history in Korea. For example, several scholars died by suicide in 1905 to protest the colonial occupation of Korea by the Japanese (Jang, 2004). In the last thirty years of the 20th Century, nearly 100 people killed themselves in South Korea as a means of political protest (Park, 2004). These fell mainly into two groups: (1) workers protesting the repression of workers and their unions by companies and by the government, and (2) students protesting the government's policies and its cooperation with the United States in the confrontation with North Korea. Some of the protest suicides left suicide notes.

Park (2004) noted that these suicides were not impulsive acts. Sometimes their suicide notes were written a few days before the actual suicide, and the protest suicide was mentioned in the diaries of the suicides months earlier. The decisions were reached after a great deal of reflection and soul-searching. Protest suicides do not appear undertaken by people with psychiatric disorders, but rather are the product of mature reasoning. Since the aim of the protest suicides is to change society, the suicides may be classified as altruistic in Durkheim's (1897) system. Park observed that the suicide notes typically involved a challenge or a message to one's own group, as well as to the powerful group against which they were struggling, a message that more should be done to overcome the wrongs and injustices.

Two samples of notes from protest suicides in South Korea were obtained from the period 1975 to 2003, a period during which South Korea was mostly ruled by authoritarian military leaders. There were 15 notes from workers and 16 from students. The majority of the suicide notes were obtained from two underground compendia (*Everlasting Lives*) compiled in 1990 and 1998 by the Ad Hoc Committee for the Preparation of a Memorial Services for the Nation's Martyrs and Victims of the Democratization Movement, a committee established in part by families of the suicides. Others were obtained from a variety of sources, including leaflets, newspapers and magazines and from the families of the suicides. These notes are from about one-third of the protest suicides taking place in South Korea from 1970-2003. Other protest suicides either did not leave notes, or their notes were not available.[46]

The two samples of notes (from the workers and the students, respectively) did not differ in sex (93% and 81% were written by men, respectively), using fire as a method for suicide (80% and 62½%, respectively), using multiple methods for suicide (33% and 31%, respectively), or leaving more than one suicide note (27% and 31%, respectively). The two samples of notes did not differ in length (292 and 411 words,

45 This chapter was co-authored with B. C. Ben Park and based on Park and Lester (2009).

46 Where possible, Ben Park visited families to request the original suicide note in order to check the content against the published version. In no case was any editorial change noted.

respectively). As expected, the workers were older than the students (mean ages 30.7 and 22.3 years, respectively).

14.1 The LIWC Analysis

Using t-tests, significant differences were identified for six variables out of the 74 variables examined, no more than would be expected on the basis of chance (see Table 14-1). The differences were in words longer than six letters (students had a higher percentage), prepositions (students had a higher percentage), words concerned with inhibition such as *block* or *constrain* (students had a higher percentage), inclusive words such as *with* and *include* (students had a higher percentage), job or work words such as *employ* and *career* (students had a lower percentage), and music words such as *tunes* and *songs* (students had a higher percentage). These differences did not seem to be psychologically meaningful.

Tab. 14.1: Differences between the suicide notes of students and workers (mean scores shown)

	students	**workers**
Words longer than 6 letters	21.9	17.2**
Prepositions	14.6	12.5*
Inhibition	0.74	0.40*
Inclusive	7.0	5.8*
Job	0.7	2.4**
Music	0.1	0.0*
Words per sentence	422.8	321.1#
First person singular	4.1	6.1#
Total first person	6.4	7.9#
Tentative	1.4	1.0#
Seeing	0.3	0.2#
School	1.4	0.4#
Leisure	0.6	1.1#
Home	0.4	1.1#
Sexual	0.3	0.1#
Eating	0.01	0.10#

* two-tailed $p < .05$, ** two-tailed $p < .01$, # trend (two-tailed $p < 0.10$)

The notes were also examined for the frequency of specific words using Microsoft Word's icon for *Find*. The students' notes were protesting against "America" more often than were the workers (62½% versus 7%) and more often against the "regime" in South Korea (75% versus 33%). The students' notes more often mentioned the "minjung" (masses) (69% versus 7%) and more often urged reunification of Korea (37½% versus 7%).

The groups of notes from students and workers did not differ in whether they were addressed to parents (37½% versus 40%, respectively), mentioned being sorry (19% versus 27%), asked for forgiveness (12½% versus 20%), mentioned being an undutiful son or daughter (25% versus 33%), referred to suicide in some way (death, act, leaving, etc.) (69% versus 60%, respectively), or used a more direct word for death (25% versus 20%). As for the emotions expressed, the students and workers did not differ in the mention of any emotion (62% versus 40%, respectively), or anger (6% versus 20%), anguish (0% versus 13%) and sadness (25% versus 13%).

Thus, the notes of these two groups, students and workers, were similar in the themes expressed. However, the focus of the notes was clearly different. The students were protesting national causes and expressed opposition to the government and America and urged reunification of the Korean peninsular. In contrast, the workers were protesting the practices of their companies and fighting for the rights of the workers. It seems that the tradition of protest suicide in Confucianism has a unique character in modern Korean society. The students appeared to be acting on broad principles based on abstract ideas of national identity opposition to the government. In contrast, the suicide notes of the laborers expressed feelings of injustice existing in the context of their group, and their suicides seemed to invite emotional sympathy from others.

The differences found in these two groups of protest suicide notes may also be an indication of differences in social class. A sense of moral duty, associated with reforming zeal and obligations reflects the elitism that exists among the students. The idea of revenge against their employers, which is more common in the suicide notes from the workers, reflects more context-dependent concerns and is designed to evoke sympathetic reactions from others.

Overall, it seems that, rather than the individual propensity, the protest suicide of both students and workers was affected more by the historical time in which intense socio-political conflict was imposed upon these individuals whose personal identities were acutely disturbed. The historical legacy of protest suicide in Korea and shared collective ideals (i.e., democratization for the *minjung*, justice and equality for the workers, and reunification of the nation) appear to serve a significant normative force behind the decision to act. These protest suicides seem to have placed a high value on identification with the larger group, and it seems that protest suicide may be viewed as a sacrificial death based on a decision to act demanded by the collective conscience, in the context of a conflict-laden socio-political struggle. If they had been able to develop a more meaningful personal identity that enabled them to sustain enduring attachment to others, they might not have seen their cause as more important than their life.

Part III: **Studies Of Other Written Materials**

15 Studies of Poems

Several poets have died by suicide, and so it of interest to explore whether changes occurred in their poems as they day of their death grew closer.

15.1 Sara Teasdale[47]

Sara Teasdale (August 8, 1884 – January 29, 1933) was an American poet from Missouri. After her father died in 1914, Sara married a local businessman, but the marriage was one of convenience. Sara was frigid and used mild illnesses as an excuse to get away from him. Sara divorced him in 1929. From that time on, she lived alone in a hotel, with only visits from a close friend to cheer her up. She became depressed and worried about her health and her finances. She killed herself in her bathtub with an overdose of sedatives.

Drake (1979) noted that four major women poets of the 19th Century (Emily Bronte, Christina Rossetti, Emily Dickinson and Elizabeth Barrett Browning until she was forty) were all recluses like Sara. All four belonged to very close family units which fulfilled their desires for affection and intellectual stimulation. Sara ventured out more than some of her predecessors but continually retreated into seclusion because of her "illnesses," becoming almost a total recluse by the end of her life.

The Victorian era encouraged women in the creative arts but undermined their self-confidence. They were allowed to dabble, but they were not supposed to achieve. When they did write poetry, they wrote mostly about love and the desire to submit to the ideal lover. However, it was not always easy to find this in their own lives. They often ended up renouncing love for men and substituting an attraction to death. They frequently had mysterious physical weaknesses and chronic ill health, a neurotic way of resolving the conflict between their personal desires and the conventions imposed upon them by the society.

The present analysis examined the poems of Sara Teasdale (Teasdale, 1938) for changes in their content from her first collection (in 1907) to her final (and 7th) collection (in 1933). Each of the 317 poems was labeled by the year of the collection that they appeared in (from 1907 to 1933). There were 25 significant correlations out of 74 examined, significantly more than would be expected by chance (see Table 15-1). The two most interesting trends were: (1) a decrease in positive emotions and feelings over time, and (2) fewer references to herself and to others. There was no change in the use of words related to death, but there were fewer references to religion and to physical states and functions, the body, sexual activities and sleep. There was a decrease in references to the present and an increase in references to the future.

47 This section was co-authored with Stephanie McSwain.

Tab. 15.1: Correlations over time for the poems of Sara Teasdale, numbered by the year of the book in which they appeared

	Pearson r
Word count	-0.15**
Words per sentence	0.15**
Unique words	0.19**
Words long than 6 letters	0.13*
Pronouns	-0.15**
First person singular	-0.16**
Total first person	-0.15**
Total third person	-0.13*
Negations	0.14*
Affect	-0.15**
Positive emotions	-0.13*
Positive feelings	-0.18**
Social processes	-0.12*
Time	0.13*
Present tense verbs	-0.12*
Future tense verbs	0.16**
Space	0.17**
Up	0.20**
Motion	0.14*
Occupation	0.11*
Religion	-0.16**
Physical states	-0.34**
Body	-0.26**
Sexual	-0.23**
Sleep	-0.14*
Prepositions	0.10#
Senses	-0.09#
Other references to people	-0.10#
Metaphysical issues	-0.11#

* two-tailed p < .05, ** two-tailed p < .01, # trend (two-tailed p < 0.10)

Some of these trends have psychodynamic significance. For example, there was a decline in positive emotions and feelings in the later poems, in contrast to the increase in positive emotions in Katie's diary (Chapter 3), and the poems also became more impersonal, with fewer references to herself and to others.

Poems are crafted to a much great extent than diary entries and letters, and so much of the "personal" content may be eliminated or changed in line with the structure of the poem. It is to be expected, therefore, that poems will be less influenced by the state of mind of the poet than would be diaries and letters.

15.2 Sylvia Plath[48]

Sylvia Plath (October 27, 1932 – February 11, 1963) was an American poet who died at the age of thirty in 1963 in England by putting her head in the gas oven. At the time of her death, her husband, the British poet Ted Hughes, had left Sylvia for another woman, leaving Sylvia with two small children and living in an apartment in London. Sylvia probably had a bipolar affective disorder (manic-depressive disorder), and in the final months of her life experienced a creative burst, writing many new poems.

The Collected Poems (Plath, 1981) has the poems organized by the date of writing. The selection of 50 "juvenilia" poems was discarded. The remaining poems start in 1956 and extend through to 1963. The 224 poems were labeled by the year of writing. Correlations over time were carried out for all 224 poems, for the 69 poems written in the last year of her life and for the 12 poems written in the last month of her life. In addition, the poems written in 1962 were compared by means of t-tests with those written in 1963.

15.2.1 1956-1963

For all 224 poems written as an adult, there were 29 significant correlations (see Table 15-2). Over this eight year period, positive feelings increased (including optimism) but so did negative emotions. References to herself and to "you" increased. References to the present and future increased, but there no changes in references to the past. References to religion, death and metaphysical issues increased.

15.2.2 The Last Year

Fifteen significant correlations were identified for the poems over the last year of her life, more than would be expected by chance (see Table 15-2). The poems got shorter, but with more words per sentence. There were more unique words and fewer question

48 This section was co-authored with Stephanie McSwain.

marks and words found in dictionaries. Positive emotions increased, but there were fewer words dealing with cognitive mechanisms and insight. There was less focus on the present and more focus on the body and eating. There were no changes in words related to death, religion or metaphysical issues.

Tab. 15.2: The results of the LIWC analysis of Sylvia Path's poems

	By year	Over last	Over last	1962 versus 1963[49] means	
	n=224	year n=69	month n=12	1962	1963
Word count	0.15*	-0.30*	-0.25	284.3	129.4*
Words per sentence	-0.57**	0.43**	-0.18	12.2	17.0**
Question marks	0.36**	-0.30*	0.02	0.94	0.42#
Unique words	-0.53**	0.41**	0.01	64.4	72.6**
Words in the dict.	0.62**	-0.27*	-0.10	67.3	63.8*
Words with 6+ letters	-0.29**	0.02	-0.56#		
Pronouns	0.47**	-0.36**	-0.32	11.9	7.7**
First person singular	0.35**	-0.11	-0.47		
First person plural	-0.09	-0.21#	0.39		
Total first person	0.29**	-0.16	-0.42		
Total second person	0.24**	-0.16	-0.17	1.9	0.7**
Negations	0.22**	0.05	-0.44		
Assent	0.01	0.01	-	0.08	0.00#
Articles	0.43**	0.24#	0.18		
Prepositions	-0.41**	0.30*	0.27	10.3	12.7**
Numbers	0.08	0.23#	0.24		
Affect	0.13#	0.06	0.20		
Positive emotions	0.05	0.24*	0.04		
Positive feelings	0.23**	-0.01	-0.21		
Optimism	-0.17**	0.11	0.18		
Negative emotions	0.14*	-0.16	0.20		
Anxiety	0.12#	-0.08	0.49		
Cognitive processes	0.06	-0.38**	-0.20		
Causation	-0.10	-0.23#	-0.16	0.43	0.18*
Insight	0.10	-0.24*	0.08		
Discrepancies	0.05	-0.21#	-0.23		

49 Using the t-test for unequal variances.

continued Tab. 15.2: The results of the LIWC analysis of Sylvia Path's poems

	By year n=224	Over last year n=69	Over last month n=12	1962 versus 1963[49] means 1962	1963
Inhibition	-0.14*	-0.18	-0.34		
Certainty	0.06	0.24*	-0.27		
Seeing	-0.12#	-0.08	-0.30		
Social processes	0.12#	-0.11	0.15	7.4	4.9*
Other refs to people	0.10	-0.21#	0.30	5.1	3.2#
Friends	0.01	-0.15	-	0.11	0.00**
Humans	0.08	0.20#	-0.23		
Past tense verbs	-0.12#	-0.16	-0.12		
Present tense verbs	0.57**	-0.47**	0.29	9.0	6.8**
Future tense verbs	0.19**	0.09	-0.08		
Up	-0.12#	0.12	0.26		
Exclusive	0.03	-0.18	-0.66*		
Occupations	-0.14*	0.05	0.26		
Job	-0.14*	-0.08	-	0.13	0.00**
Sports	0.09	0.24*	-0.12		
TV	-0.02	-0.08	-	0.03	0.00*
Money	-0.29**	-0.17	-	0.13	0.00**
Metaphysical issues	0.31**	0.08	-0.15		
Religion	0.17**	0.08	-0.48		
Death	0.29*	0.04	0.29		
Physical states	0.16*	0.24*	-0.14		
Body	0.14*	0.22#	-0.32		
Sexual	0.15*	0.06	-0.28		
Eating	-0.02	0.27*	0.14		
Sleep	-0.10	-0.19	-0.13	0.18	0.05#
Grooming	0.18**	0.03	0.31		

* two-tailed p < .05, ** two-tailed p < .01, # trend (two-tailed p < 0.10)

15.2.3 The Last Month

Interestingly, over the last month of her life (see Table 15-2), only one significant trend was found (fewer words of exclusion over time), but one significant correlation in 74 analyses is not a reliable finding.

15.2.4 1963 Versus 1962

Fifteen significant differences were found in the poems written in 1963 versus 1962. The poems in the past month of her life were shorter, with more unique words and fewer dictionary words. There were fewer references to "you" and fewer words relevant to causation. Positive and negative emotions did not change. There were fewer references to others and to friends and less emphasis on the present but no changes in words relevant to religion, death or metaphysical issues.

15.2.5 Discussion

It has been argued that Plath had a bipolar affective disorder and that she was in a manic phase while writing her final poems. There are many poems from this period, and they are not as well-crafted as her earlier poems. The major trends toward the end of her life were shorter poems, with more unique words and fewer words found in dictionaries. Over the final year, positive emotions became more common, as with Katie's diary (see Chapter 3). There was less emphasis on the present but no changes in words related to death. However, over her life as a poet overall, references to death increased and both positive and negative emotions increased, as did self-references. Unlike the findings in the previous chapter for Sara Teasdale, the changes in Sylvia Plath's poems have more psychodynamic significance, and this is probably a result of Plath's focus on much more personal issues than the poems of Teasdale.

15.3 Weldon Kees[50]

Weldon Kees (February 24, 1914 to July 18, 1955) was an American poet who also painted and wrote novels and short stories. On July 19, 1955, his car was found abandoned on the Golden Gate Bridge. There was no suicide note, and no one saw him jump. When friends went to his apartment, his sleeping bag and bank-books were missing. He was presumed to have killed himself.

50 This section was co-authored by Leah Henderson.

Kees had recently divorced his wife who was an alcoholic and who had psychotic tendencies. In the last few years of his life, Kees showed symptoms of mild mania and abandoned what he was good at (writing poetry) in order to become involved in other projects, few of which came to fruition. In order to keep up with hectic life, he took amphetamines to stay awake and sedatives to go to sleep. In the last few days of his life, he talked about a friend of either jumping off the Golden Gate Bridge or going to Mexico.

Kees wrote three books of poems: *The last man* in 1943, *The fall of the Magician* in 1947, and *Poems 1947-1954* in 1954. In *The collected poems of Weldon Kees* (Justice, 2003), there are also 16 poems from the 1940s and 1950s, never collected before, placed in rough chronological order. For the LIWC analysis, each poem in the published books was labeled by the book (1, 2 and 3) and all 107 poems were analyzed by the LIWC program and correlated with the book number that the poems were in. Second, the 16 extra poems were numbered by chronological order and their LIWC scores correlated with this number. The results are shown in Table 15-3.

It can be seen that 17 correlations over all 107 of his published poems were statistically significant, but only five over the 16 extra poems. Over the books of his poems, the poems got longer, had more references to himself and fewer to social processes, had fewer references to negative emotions, especially anxiety and to a lesser extent anger, and fewer references to the future. These trends were also apparent to some extent in the 16 extra poems.

It is interesting that in some of the analyses of the present book negative emotions decrease over time and sometimes positive emotions increase over time. We will explore in the final chapter where these trends appeared and whether there is any pattern that can be discerned.

15.4 Landis Everson[51]

Landis Everson was born in Colorado in 1926. He finished a Master's degree at Columbia University in 1951, moved to California and wrote poems which were published. He then stopped writing for 43 years, turning to painting for ten years and then remodeling and renovating houses. His next poem, published in 2004, was his first publication since 1962. He published his first book of poems and in 2005 received a prize for the best first book of poems by a poet over 50. He killed himself with a firearm at the age of 81 on November 17, 2007, after suffering a stroke which left him unable to write.

51 This section was co-authored with Stephanie McSwain.

Tab. 15.3: Correlations over time for Weldon Kees's poems

	Correlations by book (1, 2, 3) n = 107	**Correlations for the final 16 poems (1-16) n =16**
Word count	0.26**	-0.21
Unique words	-0.20*	-0.08
Words long than 6 letters	-0.27**	-0.61*
First person singular	0.21*	0.51*
Total first person	0.20*	0.29
Negation	-0.25**	-0.09
Articles	0.20*	0.29
Prepositions	0.24*	0.52*
Affect	-0.29**	-0.29
Negative emotions	-0.25**	-0.40
Anxiety	-0.28**	-0.30
Cognitive processes	-0.21*	-0.58*
Senses	-0.22*	0.18
Hearing	-0.20*	0.17
Social processes	-0.30**	0.01
Communication	-0.25**	0.12
Inclusive	0.29**	-0.01
Motion	0.08	0.61*
Words per sentence	-0.16#	-0.25
Total third person	-0.16#	0.12
Optimism	-0.10	-0.44#
Anger	-0.10	-0.44#
Insight	-0.18#	-0.37
Tentative	-0.07	-0.49#
Seeing	-0.18#	0.14
Other references to people	-0.19#	-0.02
Time	0.18#	0.47#
Future	-0.17#	-0.41
Music	-0.17#	-0.15
Death	-0.17#	-0.32

* two-tailed p < .05, ** two-tailed p < .01, # trend (two-tailed p < 0.10)

Tab. 15.4: A comparison between the 9 early poems and 66 later poems of Landis Everson (mean scores shown)

	Early poems	Later poems
Negations	0.82	2.07*
Anxiety	0.46	0.16*
Tentative	1.02	1.70*
Past tense verbs	1.81	3.15**
Inclusive	7.69	5.30**
Occupations	0.41	1.04**
School	0.03	0.30**
Home	0.10	0.32*
Word count	395.11	132.32#
Unique words	64.21	70.51#
Humans	1.06	0.29#
Sleep	0.61	0.19#

* two-tailed p < .05, ** two-tailed p < .01, # trend (two-tailed p < 0.10)

Everson's poems, therefore, were written in two widely separated eras (Everson, 2006). The 9 early poems are much longer than the later 66 poems, which makes it difficult to compare the two sets reliably. As a result of this, since the variances of the scores for the two samples were not similar, the alternative t-test was used. The results are shown in Table 15-4. Twelve significant differences were found. From a psychodynamic perspective, the interesting differences are a reduction in anxiety in the later poems, fewer references to people, and a greater emphasis on the past. But the differences are not as extensive or as relevant for understanding Kees's state of mind as those identified in the section above on Sylvia Plath's poems.

15.5 Katie's Poems[52]

In Chapter 3, the diary left by a young woman, Katie, who killed herself was analyzed. Katie also wrote poems and dated some of them by the year in which they were written. These dated poems cover a four year period, and Katie died in the middle of the following year. The 83 dated poems were labeled by the year in which they were written and analyzed using the LIWC program. The correlations over the four years

52 This section was co-authored with Stephanie McSwain.

(labeled 1, 2, 3 and 4) are shown in Table 15-5. Eleven significant changes were found and six trends.

Most of these poems were written by Katie prior to the period covered by her diary. Unlike the results for the diary, these were no changes in emotions over time for these poems. References to death and to religion did not change. There was less emphasis on the present and future over time, but no increase in references to the past. Katie seemed less concerned with cognitive processes and insight over time in these poems (words such as cause, know and ought and think, know and consider).

Tab. 15.5.: Correlations over the four years for 83 poems by Katie, labelled by the year each was written.

	Correlation
Words per sentence	0.23*
First person plural	-0.27*
Total third person	0.30**
Cognitive processes	-0.25*
Other references to people	0.24*
Present tense verbs	-0.32**
Future tense verbs	-0.31**
Up	0.26*
Achievement	-0.24*
Leisure	0.24*
Swearing	0.31**
Words in the dictionary	-0.21#
Insight	-0.20#
Social processes	0.21#
Home	0.19#
Sports	0.19#
Body	0.22#

* two-tailed $p < .05$, ** two-tailed $p < .01$, # trend (two-tailed $p < 0.10$)

15.6 Discussion

This study of the poems of these poets who died by suicide did not identify as many interesting trends over time as their deaths came closer as did the studies of diaries. As mentioned above, perhaps the crafting of poems and the application of rules of sound and meter impair the direct and indirect communication of psychodynamic factors in the words and sentences written by these poets. Alternatively other techniques of studying poems (other than the LIWC) may prove more fruitful.

16 Studies of Letters

I have obtained several series of letters written by people in the months prior to the death by suicide. The present chapter explores whether trends can be found in these letters over time as the day of death grew closer.

16.1 Letters from a Young Man to a Friend[53]

Suicides often write ordinary letters to friends and family members. It would be of interest if these letters showed trends as the individual gets closer in time to the act of suicide. There has been no published study on such personal letters written before, and this chapter will apply the LIWC technique to study a series of personal letters written before an individual's suicidal death.

The materials consisted of 19 letters written by a young man to a friend covering a two-year period prior to his death by suicide. There was a suicide note, but this note was not included in the analysis. His friend kept these letters and gave them to the young man's mother. These notes are not suicide notes, but ordinary letters written to one person. However, like a diary, the successive letters are written closer and closer in time to the writer's death, and so they allow an examination of whether any trends can be ascertained as the young man approached the time of his death. The first letter was written 24 months before his death and the 19th letter 15 days before his death at the age of 20. When he died, the young man was attending college and playing for the college baseball team.

Tab. 16.1: Correlations over time (the notes were numbered in sequence from 1 to 19) and the content of the 19 letters

	Pearson r
Words per sentence	0.72**
Pronouns	-0.49*
Humans	0.59**
Time	0.48*
Affect	-0.45#
Negative emotions	-0.39#
Anxiety	-0.40#
Causation	-0.39#
Eating	0.42#

* two-tailed p < .05, ** two-tailed p < .01, # trend (two-tailed p < 0.10)

53 This section is based on Barnes, et al. (2007).

Trends in the letters were examined by correlating the number of the letter in the sequence (from 1 to 19) with the scores obtained by each letter for each of the 76 categories. The correlation coefficients are shown in Table 16-1. Only four correlations were significant: as the letters are closer to the time of young man's suicide, the words per sentence increased, as did words related to humans and time, while the use of pronouns decreased. Five further correlations showed non-significant trends. As the letters came closer to the suicide of the young man, there was a decrease in the proportion of words related to emotions in general, negative emotions, anxiety and causation, and an increase in the proportion words associated with eating.

Eight trends were noted by Pennebaker and Stone (2004) in their analysis of Katie's diary (see Chapter 3), one of which were replicated in these letters: the proportion of negative emotion words declined. Thus, the letters sounded somewhat more positive as the death of this young man came closer inasmuch as mention of negative emotions declined. However, mention of positive emotions did not increase. As noted in earlier chapters, this decrease in negative emotion words suggests that, as a person draws closer to the time of their suicide, their mood may improve. The current study, as well as Katie's diary, suggests that the trend may be long-term (over the course of months) rather than merely short-term (in the few days prior to the death by suicide).

It is clear that interesting trends relevant to the psychodynamics of this young man's decision can be gained from an examination of this sequence of letters. The next three sections examine three other series of letters which are not as useful. The first series is from a young woman to her sister, but they stop several months prior to her death. Two further series are letters from Vincent van Gogh to his sister and to his brother, both of which are somewhat business oriented.

16.2 Letters from a Young Woman to her sister

Kramer (2002) presented the life story of a young woman, Clara, who killed herself. Kramer used personal documents donated to the library at Rutgers University, including 90 letters written to her sister in the year prior to her suicide. This section will describe some of the stepping stones in Clara's life and subject her letter to an analysis using the LIWC. The following biographical details are based on information in the paper published by Kramer.

16.2.1 Clara's Life

Clara, born in 1917 in Pennsylvania, was raised in a devout Roman Catholic family and briefly considered becoming a nun. In adolescence, she began to question the rigid beliefs of the church, and attended the New Jersey College for Women (later Douglas College at Rutgers University), graduating in 1938.

Her parents were from Slovenia and had moved to an ethnic enclave in New Jersey. Her father worked in factories, but he was often out of work like many men during the Great Depression. Her mother worked occasionally as a seamstress in New York City. The first born, Elsie, was four years older than Clara. A son came later but drowned in a well at the age of three. From a reading of Clara's high-school diary and a short-story she wrote, Kramer felt that Clara had unresolved grief over this loss.

The family considered Clara to be intellectually gifted, and Elsie, who took a maternal role with Clara, helped support her through college. After graduating from college with honors, Clara earned a Master's Degree in English literature from Columbia University. She was socially active and well-liked throughout her high school and college years.

After graduating, she worked as a secretary for publishers in New York City and commuted there for six years. However, in 1946 at the age of 28, she had a nervous breakdown which she attributed to overwork and a painful affair with a married man. She retreated to her home with symptoms of depression as well as medical problems (headaches, a thyroid condition and cessation of her period). Despite this, she returned to work in June 1946. In November 1946, Clara went to Miami to regain her health, make some money and write a semi-autobiographical novel, but she returned home in July 1947 with her goals unmet. At home, she taught at a local business college, but killed herself by hanging in September 1947.

Kramer noted that Clara's depressions began in eighth grade, at which time she complained of an unbearable fatigue and a sense of futility. From her diary from those years, it seems that, although she appeared to others to be fine, inwardly she suffered from low self-esteem and vacillated between feelings of self-confidence and feelings of worthlessness and despair. Her depressions continued throughout high school. Clara sought reinforcement from others and showed a tendency to strive for perfection, sometimes to the point of exhaustion.

Clara searched for a meaning in her life, sometimes finding this in intense religious convictions, but losing it during periods of doubt and alienation. In her letters home (which extend from November 15, 1946, to June 19, 1947), Clara seems to be unrealistically reassured that her ordeal was over. She seems convinced that her novel will win a prize and bring her wealth. She sounds optimistic about the future, but doubts appear toward of the last of the letters. After months of superficial chit-chat to her sister about her secretarial jobs, clothes and the money she owes her sister and parents, she seems to succumb to fatigue and depression again. What I found surprising, given her attempt to recover from her "nervous breakdown" and her impending suicide just a few months hence, is how superficial the content of the letters is.

Kramer felt, quite reasonably, that something must have happened in those last few months in Miami to trigger the return to depression and despair, but there is nothing in the letters or elsewhere to indicate what it might be. Kramer reported speculation from informants that there was another thwarted love affair, but there is no concrete information about this and nothing about it in the letters.

Kramer focused her analysis of Clara on the issue of religion and spirituality, especially the splitting between seeing "religion as the finest thing in the world" to having a "sense of futility, and a strong aversion to religion – as strong an aversion against religion as the desire for it had been."

Clara was the second-born, and yet she was seen as the gifted one who was going to succeed, a role typically assigned to the first-born. She came from a lower-class family and was going to be the first educated member.[54] (In earlier Catholic families, the eldest son became the achiever and the second-born son a priest. In Clara's family there were two daughters rather than sons, and Clara at one point wanted to become a nun.) She experienced this pressure to succeed academically, yet the society still discriminated against women. Clara went to a "college for women" and then worked as a secretary despite her Masters Degree. She aspired to teach – even in Miami she toyed with the idea of teaching at the local colleges – but instead worked as a typist. Today, if she willingly chose to take an academic route, she might have finished a doctorate and become a college professor, but such a path was more difficult in the 1930s, especially if you were taking this route because your parents had chosen it for you. Thus, while Kramer focuses on internal religious conflict and a search for meaning, it seems to me that the parents' conditions of worth for this young girl possibly led to her taking a path that was forced upon her and would not have been her first choice.

Of course, we lack a great deal of information about her life. What were her parents like? Was there love or abuse in the family? How did Clara's father handle the Great Depression and his periods out of work? What were the circumstances of her younger brother's death, who was there when he drowned, and how did the family handle this?[55] Had this boy survived, would he rather than Clara have borne his parents' expectations of the American dream? When did she first date boys, who were her first loves, and what were the details of the affair with the married man?

Her letters to her sister in the months prior to her death are full of concerns over money, even trivial amounts (often characteristic of those who grew up during the Great Depression) and a concern with the superficial aspects of life – dresses, getting praise from her boss, and how much more mature she is than her friends. Had she not been labeled as the academically-gifted daughter, she might well have ended up in the standard role as housewife and mother, concerned with the decoration of the house and the appearance of her children, combined with conventional religious adherence. But her education led her to think, to question and to aspire, all of which made the housewife and mother role impossible. In several of her letters, she talks of her desire to marry a wealthy man, as long as he wasn't Jewish!

---

54 I was struck by her anti-semitism in the letters to her sister. Although not unusual, especially in the 1930s in America, it also suggests rigid lower-class values in her Catholic parents.

55 I am reminded here of the incredible impact of the death of Vincent van Gogh's elder brother prior to Vincent's birth and the impact that this had on him through the reactions of his parents to this loss.

The LIWC analysis, of course, will not shed any light on the speculations of Kramer or myself. Rather, it will identify trends, if any, over the ninety letters (numbered 1 to 90) to her sister over the seven months (November 15, 1946 to June 19, 1947) prior to her suicide three months later in September 1947.

The LIWC analysis (see Table 16-2) identified 17 significant linear trends over the seven months, significantly more than would be expected by chance in 74 comparisons. Clara made fewer references to her self over time and also fewer to her family. Negative emotions became more common, including anxiety and sadness. There were more words concerned with cognitive mechanisms and insight, fewer references to the past and more to the present. Clara also showed less concern with her body and associated processes, such as eating and sleeping.

Tab. 16.2: Changes in the 90 letters (numbered 1 to 90) from Clara over time

	Correlation
First person singular	-0.25*
Total first person	-0.29**
Total second person	0.25*
Numbers	-0.24*
Negative emotions	0.26*
Sad	0.25*
Cognitive processes	0.35**
Insight	0.22*
Tentative	0.40**
Feeling	0.26*
Family	-0.22*
Past tense verbs	-0.23*
Present tense verbs	0.25*
Motion	-0.37**
Physical states	-0.30**
Eating	-0.31**
Sleep	-0.21*
Anxiety	0.20#
Certainty	-0.18#
Leisure	-0.19#

* two-tailed p < .05, ** two-tailed p < .01, # trend (two-tailed p < 0.10)

Previous studies in this book have shown a decrease in negative emotions for some suicides and an increase in positive emotions. It must be remembered here that, for Clara, the letters end three months before she killed herself and, therefore, the letters do not give any clues as to what changes might have occurred in these last three months of her life. However, it seems that, for Clara, her mood was worsening as time passed. Any additional set-backs in the final three months may have exacerbated an already suicidogenic state of mind.

16.3 Letters from Vincent Van Gogh to his Sister

As we saw above, in a series of letters from a young man who died by suicide to a friend, there were trends over time including a decrease in words indicating negative emotions and an increase in death words. There was a decrease in the proportion of words concerned with negative emotions and with anxiety and an increase in the number of words per sentence. These trends were not replicated in the analysis of the letters from a young woman to her sister.

The letters of Vincent Van Gogh (1853-1890), the artist, are available online (www.vggallery.com), and the present study used the LIWC to examine the 22 letters (numbered 1 to 22) written by Van Gogh to his sister Wil from 1887 to June 12, 1890, just prior to his suicide.

Tab. 16.3: Correlations over time for the letters (numbered 1 to 22) of Vincent Van Gogh to his sister

	Pearson r
Words longer than 6 letters	-0.51*
Negations	-0.48*
Anxiety	0.48*
Seeing	0.43*
Time	0.44*
Past tense verbs	0.45*
School	-0.49*
Music	-0.46*
Word count	-0.39#
First person singular	0.39#
Insight	0.39#
Tentative	-0.41#
Down	0.38#

* two-tailed $p < .05$, ** two-tailed $p < .01$, # trend (two-tailed $p < 0.10$)

There were eight significant trends over time, from the 1st to the 22nd letter (see Table 16-3). The proportion of long words decreased, as did the proportion of negations, words concerned with school, and words concerned with music, while the proportion of anxiety words increased, as well as words concerned with seeing, time and the past. However, eight significant correlations out of 74 examined is only slightly greater than would be expected by chance alone. Furthermore, the trends identified here do not resemble those found above and so may be unique to this set of letters rather than characteristic of the letters of suicides in general, except that, like the letters from Clara to her sister, anxiety-related words increased over time.

16.4 Letters from Vincent Van Gogh to his Brother

As noted above, Vincent van Gogh's letters are available on the website www.vggallery.com. The 43 letters to his brother Theo, written in the last year of van Gogh's life (numbered 1 to 43), were analyzed using the LIWC program for changes over time. In addition, the five letters written in the last month of his life were analyzed in a similar fashion and also compared with the remaining 38 letters from that last year.[56]

Very few changes occurred over the last year of Van Gogh's life in these letters (see Table 16-4) – only eight significant trends out of 74 possibilities. The letters grew shorter, had more unique words, had fewer negations, had more social words (with more references to family and others), fewer words associated with feelings and fewer references to time. None of these trends appear to have much psychological significance.

There were only five letters in the last month of Van Gogh's life, and so significant trends are difficult to identify. Only two appeared – there were fewer words related to anxiety and more related to occupation over time. The letters written in the last month were compared to those written in the prior eleven months. In the last month, the letters were shorter, had more social words and fewer time words, along with fewer school words and eating words. Again, these differences do not seem to have much psychological significance.

These analyses of letters written by Vincent van Gogh to his siblings do not seem to provide any psychodynamic insights into his state of mind, and a perusal of the letters indicates that they are rather impersonal and concerned mainly with the paintings on which he was working.

56 t-tests for unequal variances were used because of the small sample size for letters written in the month prior to his suicide.

16.5 Discussion

The first two studies in this chapter on letters were from ordinary people in the modern era and provided some interesting insights. The older and more formal letters from Vincent van Gogh to his siblings provided little of interest. It is clear, then, that the source and type of letter is critical in the insights that they give us into the suicidal mind.

Tab. 16.4: Van Gogh: Letters to his brother

	Last year (numbered 1-43)	Last month (numbered 1-5)	Rest of year means	Last month means[57]
Word count	-0.54**	-0.18	1076	504**
Question marks	0.22	0.08	0.16	0.48#
Unique words	0.53**	-0.02	40.5	51.1#
Abbreviations	0.03	-	0.01	0.00#
Pronouns	0.23	0.07	12.8	15.0#
Total second person	0.21	0.08	2.1	3.4#
Negations	-0.35*	-0.42		
Numbers	0.29#	-0.25		
Negative emotions	0.06	-0.67	1.1	1.7#
Anxiety	0.21	-0.99**		
Inhibition	-0.07	0.87#		
Feeling	-0.36*	0.56		
Social processes	0.33*	0.06	6.8	9.2*
Other refs to people	0.34*	0.03	4.7	6.3*
Friends	0.10	0.00	0.12	0.04#
Family	0.32*	-0.38		
Time	-0.32*	-0.59	4.4	3.0**
Inclusive	-0.27#	-0.82#	7.0	5.8#
Occupations	-0.10	0.99**		
School	-0.17	0.49	0.35	0.09**
Eating	-0.12	-	0.05	0.00**

* two-tailed p < .05, ** two-tailed p < .01, # trend (two-tailed p < 0.10)

57 t-tests for unequal variances were used.

17 A Blog From a Murder-Suicide

Blogs are web pages that are frequently updated, containing current and archived text-based posts. Many blogs are interactive in that visitors to the site can leave comments. Setting up blogs has been facilitated by the development of hosting sites and software applications to facilitate individuals setting up and maintaining a blog. There have been a number of studies already investigating blogs and guidelines for conducting such research (Hookway, 2008). For example, Stefanone and Jang (2008) surveyed bloggers and found that the traits of extraversion and self-disclosure (as well as age, sex and education) were not related to using blogs to maintain relationships.

Clarke and van Amerom (2008) compared blogs written by women and men who identified themselves as depressed (identified by a web search for "depression blog"). Clarke and van Amermon used a qualitative content analysis and found that women were more likely to discuss psychotherapy and self-help while men were more likely to discuss pharmaceuticals and self-harm. The men preferred a medical approach, namely that depression is biologically based, while women more often expressed skepticism of this approach. Women were more likely to seek alternatives ways to treat their depression. Men more often saw their depression as a result of external events, such as strife in the world, whereas women focused more often on interpersonal relationships as the source. The blogs written by men contained more violent images and fantasies, especially suicide and self-harm. Huffaker and Calvert (2005) found that adolescent boys used emoticons more than girls, employed an active and resolute style of language and more often were homosexual.

Blogs have, of course, been used by those attempting and completing suicide and, therefore, lend themselves to qualitative and quantitative analyses. The present chapter examines a blog left by a man who engaged in a murder-suicide incident.[58]

On August 4th, 2009, George Sodini shot at 12 women at a health club in Pittsburgh, killing three, before killing himself. Sodini was a loner, 48 years old[59] and a systems analyst for a law firm. He lived in Carnegie, Pennsylvania, just a few miles from the scene of his murders. He was member of the health club and felt rejected by the women who worked out there and who paid him no attention. In his blog, he talked of his poor relationships with his family members and of having had no girl friend since 1984.

Sodini's blog was printed in full (with expletives and racial slurs deleted) by ABC News.[60] These entries extended from November 5th, 2008 to August 3rd, 2009. The 24 entries in the blog of Sodini were entered into the LIWC program and correlations calculated between content categories and (1) the month of each entry (numbered 1

---

58 This section is based on Lester (2010c).

59 Sodini was born 9/30/1960 and died 8/4/2009.

60 abcnews.go.com/print?id=8258001 accessed August 5, 2009.

to 10), (2) the sequence of the entries (numbered from 1 to 24), and (3) the number of days since the first entry.

Only two significant correlations were identified (see Table 17-1): there were fewer mentions of leisure and the home over the ten months. There were tendencies to having more references to "I" and to the self, more negations and references to friends, more words concerned with discrepancies (such as should or could) and exclusion (such as but and except), and fewer mentions of television.

Tab. 17.1: Correlations over time for the 24 blog entries

	By month n=24	By sequence n=24	Days since 1st blog
First person singular	0.36#	0.37*#	0.34#
Total first person	0.38#	0.39#	0.37#
Negations	0.38#	0.36#	0.33
Cognitive processes	0.33	0.34	0.40#
Discrepancies	0.35#	0.35#	0.35#
Friends	0.36#	0.36#	0.38#
Exclusive	0.34	0.34	0.36#
Leisure	-0.44*	-0.44*	-0.44*
Home	-0.42*	-0.41*	-0.37#
TV	-0.36#	-0.35#	-0.40#

* two-tailed p < .05, # trend (two-tailed p < 0.10)

Sodini's online blog, therefore, showed no similarities in language analyses to those found in the diaries of suicides. Of course, this case differs in sex, age, format (online blog versus diary) and action (murder-suicide versus suicide) from the diaries and letters examined in other sections of this book. More research is needed comparing the written materials (diaries, suicide notes and blogs) left by murder-suicides and by suicides.

18 The Final Words of a Suicide

As I have noted several times in earlier chapters, the mood of suicidal individuals improves in the 24 hours prior to their death based on documentation in the clinical notes for patients in psychiatric wards. Using the LIWC program, a similar trend over longer time periods (months) was noted in Katie's diary (Chapter 3) and in the letters from a young man to a friend (Chapter 16). The present chapter examines whether a similar trend would be found in the tape recordings left by a young man on the day of his suicide.[61]

18.1 Stephen

Stephen, an only child, was an excellent student in grade school but began to act out in the classroom. When he was 11-years-old, he was assessed for attention deficit disorder but was diagnosed with clinical depression accompanied by suicidal ideation. He wrote the following when he was twelve:

> There is no cure for this plague except death. I am trying to do my best at life, but there are to [sic] many bad things in the world to stop me. I want to live in heaven with God. If something deosn't [sic] love me I will die now. Let me out of the trap.

He was given medication, which was not very helpful, and placed in psychotherapy. As he entered his teenage years, his outlook on life became increasingly negative. In high school, he began to self-medicate with marijuana and at one point threatened suicide and was hospitalized. He refused to take the recommended medication.

Stephen had a stable support network of friends and remained loving and communicative with his parents for the most part. However, his behavior became more defiant and rebellious. At the time of his death (at the age of 18), he was trying to stay "clean" but was still using marijuana and dabbling with other drugs. There were two stressors in the days prior to his death. His plans to move out from his parents' home and share an apartment with a friend looked to be unfeasible, and there was a brush with the law over a possible burglary. For the two days prior to his death, Stephen stayed in his room.

The written texts and tape recordings made by Stephen were given to the me by his parents.[62] Stephen left seven journal entries starting from April 27th to September 26th, the day before he killed himself. From what he wrote, he expected that others

61 This chapter is based on Lester (2010d).

62 I thank Stephen's parents who very kindly allowed me to use the journal, letters and tape recordings discussed in this chapter.

might read these entries. One day before his, death, Stephen wrote several suicide notes, of which two remain, one addressed to his parents and one to a friend. On the day of his death, Stephen left two audio tapes for his parents.[63] The first was recorded around 12.30 pm, after which his mother came home and had a cup of tea and a chat with him, unaware that Stephen was planning his suicide. The second was recorded around 3 pm, and Stephen killed himself (using a firearm) between 4 pm and 5 pm in the woods close to his home.

In the first recording, Stephen was crying and very upset. He noted that he was scared about what he was to do and talked of his hopelessness over whether his life would improve. He cast his suicide as a way of escaping from his psychological pain. In the second recording, Stephen was calmer. He said that he was feeling a little better and that he was composed. He did not want to leave just the first tape for others to hear, but rather to leave them with a less upsetting message. Written transcripts of the two recordings were made. The LIWC program was used to analyze the content of Stephen's journal, the two suicide notes and the two recorded messages.

18.2 The Journal Entries over Time

Analysis of the seven journal entries by Stephen yielded only four significant Pearson correlations over time from the first entry to the seventh, no more than would be expected by chance. The changes involved references to numbers and time decreasing over time, and discrepancies (e.g., should or would) and exclusive words (e.g., but and except) increasing over time.. These changes do not appear to have any psychological significance.

18.3 The Journal Entries versus the Suicide Notes

A comparison of the two suicide notes written on the day prior to his death with the seven journal entries, using t-tests, identified 23 significant differences,[64] more than would be expected by chance. The suicide notes were briefer than the journal entries (means 147 versus 484 words, respectively), but with more words per sentence (13.0 versus 9.3). The suicide notes had fewer questions marks (0% versus 0.5%), fewer long words (8.7% versus 12.1%), fewer references to others (0% versus 1.6%), less anxiety (0% versus 0.3%) and anger (0% versus 1.6%), more discrepancies (would, should and could) (4.9% versus 2.0%), and fewer metaphorical references (0% versus 0.4%)

63 It should be noted Stephen had not used marijuana on the day he made the tape recordings.

64 Because the samples sizes were small (7 journal entries versus 2 written texts), t-tests for unequal variances were used.

and references to death (0% versus 0.3%). As noted in earlier chapters, it has been hypothesized that those about to kill themselves avoid references to death and suicide in order to suppress the emotions that would be aroused by focusing on suicide.

The suicide notes also had fewer words concerned with occupations and jobs, leisure, home, music, money, sexual matters, swear words, time, humans, up, down, and seeing.

18.4 The Journal Entries versus the Tape Recordings

A comparison of the seven journal entries with the content of the two recorded messages on the day of Stephen's death, using t-tests for unequal variances, identified 23 significant differences, again, more than would be expected by chance. Some of the differences probably reflect differences between a written text and spoken words. For example, the mean word count was greater in the tape recordings (1645 versus 484 words), with fewer unique words (22.6% versus 55.4%, respectively) and fewer long words (9.2% versus 12.1%). Other differences, however, seem less dependent on the medium of communication.

The tape recordings had more pronouns overall (21.6% versus 16.1%), especially references to "you" (1.6% versus 0.5%). The tape recordings had fewer references to emotions (3.9% versus 5.8%). There was no difference in positive emotions (2.5% versus 2.2%), but the tape recordings had fewer negative emotions (1.3% versus 3.6%), especially anger (0.3% versus 1.6%) and sadness (0.2% versus 0.9%).

The tape recordings explain Stephen's actions more than the journal entries: words related to cognitive mechanisms were more common (12.3% versus 7.0%) as were words related to insight (5.1% versus 2.1%) and "discrepancy" (should, would and could: 3.8% versus 2.0%). There was more focus on the present (20.4% versus 12.6%), and less concern with issues related to money (0.1% versus 0.7%), the body (0.5% versus 1.9%), sexuality (0.1% versus 0.8%) and sleeping (0.0% versus 0.4%), as well as fewer swear words (0.1% versus 1.0%).

18.5 A Comparison of the Two Tape Recordings

The final analysis compared the two recorded messages made on the day of Stephen's death, just after the noon hour and around 3 pm. The first segment had 1821 words and the second 1468. Since statistical tests are not appropriate for a comparison of two texts, content variables for which the percentage difference in words was 1% or more were identified. The second segment contained relatively more references to others (2.7% versus 0.6%), fewer negations (3.3% versus 4.9%), more positive emotions (3.1% versus 2.0%), fewer words concerned with cognitive mechanisms (11.4% versus 13.2%) and causation (0.9% versus 2.2%), and more social references (8.4%

versus 6.3%).[65] The second segment did not differ in the percentage of words related to death or religion or words related to anger, anxiety or sadness. The two segments did not differ greatly in negative emotions.

Overall, in the second segment, Stephen expressed more positive emotions. In addition, he is more concerned with others and less concerned with the reasons for his action. As noted in earlier chapter, Spiegel and Neuringer (1963) argued that a person about to die by suicide would avoid mentioning death and suicide in a suicide note, suppressing thoughts of the planned suicide. The proportion of death words was low in both segments (0.05% in the first and 0.27% in the second). The content of the second spoken communication was less concerned with explaining his action, and more concerned with others and with positive emotions. From the text analysis, this second communication would appear to be an attempt to reassure Stephen's significant others.

18.6 Discussion

This chapter has presented a case study involving the analysis of written and spoken communications of a young man who was about to kill himself. It is unique since, unlike studies of suicide notes in the past, these suicide notes and tape recorded messages were compared with material written by the same person (a diary).

Compared with the journal entries, the two suicide notes had as many negative emotions, but fewer words related to anxiety and anger. Although not statistically significant, the suicides notes contained more positive emotions but also more sadness than the journal entries. As the suicide notes did not mention of death at all, they seemed to have been written in a relatively calm state and oriented toward reassuring his parents and the good friend to whom the second note was addressed.

Compared with the journal entries, the tape recordings were much longer, contained many more references to the self and to "you" (his parents for whom the taped recordings were made), and many more words concerned with explaining his actions. The proportion of negative emotions was less in the tape recordings, and there was more focus on the present. The second recorded message had more positive emotions, more references to others, and less concern with explaining his actions as compared to the first recorded message. There seems to be, therefore, a calming trend and an improvement in mood as he approached his death. This explanation of recorded data confirms the observations made by Clements, et al. (1985) and by Keith-Spiegel and Spiegel (1967) based on the clinical notes in the files of psychiatric patients in the hours before who completed suicide while in a psychiatric institution.

65 There were also differences in prepositions and words concerned with space and exclusion to which it is difficult to ascribe psychological meaning.

19 Twitter Postings in the 24 Hours Prior to Suicide[66]

Today, with the advent of modern means for communication, suicidal individuals are using the Internet to post suicidal communications, including suicide notes and videos. Facebook, Youtube and Twitter have become popular for such communications. These differ from suicide notes in that suicide notes are meant to be read *after* the individual has died, whereas postings on the Internet are often meant to be read *before* the individual dies, and in occasional cases those reading or viewing the postings have alerted authorities and prevented the potential suicide from engaging in lethal actions (e.g., Janson, et al., 2001).

Although the diaries of suicidal individuals permit the study of the suicidal mind over time, the writings span months and even years. The present chapter examines postings made on a social networking website by a young girl in the final 24 hours prior to her death. This permits the study of the suicidal mind in the hours prior to the suicidal act.[67]

Ashley Billasano, an 18-year-old living in Texas, died by suicide[68] after sending 145 tweets in the 24 hours prior to her suicide. In these tweets, she alleged that she had been sexually abused from ages 14 to 17 by her father. She tried to bring the abuser to justice, but she had received news that her alleged abuser would not be prosecuted. After Ashley's death, her mother said that Ashley felt that the investigation into her abuse had made her feel like a suspect rather than the victim that she was. The investigating authorities were accused of being insensitive and sending her back to the home where the alleged abuse took place because they claimed that they could not remove her. Texas Child and Protective Services had conducted a five-month investigation but were unable to confirm that the abuse had taken place (CBS News, November 15, 2011). The authorities, of course, denied any wrongdoing but, after Ashley's suicide, claimed that they would look further into her allegations. However, as of March 9, 2012, no action had been taken.

On the day of her death, Ashley told her friend who usually drove her to school that she was feeling ill. From 6:44 am to 2:08 pm she issued 144 tweets. She had over 500 followers, but it is not known whether any were monitoring her that day. During the sequence of tweets, there was a break of 139 minutes after 10:42 am and another 21 minute break after 1:47 pm. No one seems to have intervened in those periods and,

66 This chapter was written with John F. Gunn III and a brief report was published by Gunn and Lester (2012).

67 The majority of the details of the case were obtained from an online article by Craig Malisow published in the Houston Press: www/houstonpress.com/content/printVersion/2901386/ accessed December 26, 2012.

68 Ashley died by asphyxiation using helium and a plastic bag, a method she had researched on YouTube and Wikipedia.

again, it is not known whether anyone knew of what was transpiring. At 2:08 pm in her last tweet, Ashley said, "Take two. I hope I get this right."[69]

Ashley came from a dysfunctional family. Ashley's mother had accused her own father of molesting her, and Ashley's grandmother had accused her own father of molesting her. Ashley's mother married two men, one of whom sexually assaulted Ashley and was sent to prison for eleven years. Ashley's mother then met a married man who was separated, and she broke into his house with intent to murder his wife. She was sent to prison, and Ashley moved in with her father.

Other noteworthy events in Ashley's life were that she nearly drowned in a bucket of water at eleven months of age. Ashley had also been the victim of bullying in 6th grade because of her weight, after which she began cutting her wrists and developed an eating disorder. She also turned to pills and marijuana in order to cope. After her mother's release from prison, Ashley was taken on outings with family members, including an uncle who was a registered sex offender and who was later arrested for abusing an 11-year-old relative. According to Ashley's grandmother, Ashley had a nervous breakdown in 2009, after which her father obtained psychiatric treatment for her and transferred her to a charter school. There she made friends but continued to cut, and her eating disorder switched from anorexia to bulimia. She had a series of mini-romances and confessed to her friends that she had lost her virginity around age 14[70]. She had a serious romance with a young boy who apparently found out that Ashley's father was sexually abusing her. Malisow, the Houston Press reporter, could not get this boy to talk to him, and so Malisow notes that this information has not been confirmed. The boy ended the relationship. Ashley apparently told her friends that her father had caught her with drugs and blackmailed her into performing oral sex, but her friends were never sure how much of what Ashley told them was true.[71]

At her new school, she made a good friend and apparently told this friend that her father used to rent her out to his friends. Toward the end of her life, Ashley had reconnected with her boy-friend, but the relationship had broken up again, and she then received the news that no charges would be brought against her father. Ashley tried to obtain some counseling, but there was no insurance to pay for it. Ashley had been looking forward to a part in the school production of *Hairspray*, but her poor grades meant that she probably would not be allowed to participate.

After Ashley's suicide, her twitter account was closed, making retrieval of the original posts impossible. However, using an Internet search engine, the twitter posts were found reproduced in other websites and downloaded for the present analysis. News articles related to the suicide were found to contain quotes from the twitter

69 In her first tweet on the night before the series of 144 tweets the next day, she says that she failed in an earlier suicide attempt.

70 In one of her tweets, she says she was sixteen and that it was a rape.

71 In her tweets, Ashley implies that her father watched her have sex with other men.

postings, which matched the reproduced twitter postings, leading to the conclusion that the twitter postings downloaded were accurate.

The first analysis analyzed all 145 twitter postings, labeled from 1 to 145. For the second and third analyses, since Twitter postings are brief (limited to 140 characters), the postings were combined. Postings made within seconds of each other (for example, three postings made at 9:45 pm, two postings made at 10:10 pm, and so on) were combined into single postings and, next, postings made within the same hour (for example, all posts from 10:00 pm to 10:59 pm) were combined for two separate analyses. The Pearson correlations are shown in Table 19-1.

Tab. 19.1: Correlations for Twitter postings

	Correlations over postings		
	Individual Postings n=145 r	Postings Combined by minute n=75 r	Postings Combined by hour n=6 r
Word count	.55***	.23*	.24
Words per sentence	.32***	-.28*	-.11
Unique words	-.38***	-.18	-.27
Words longer than 6 letters	-.04	-.04	-.90*
Pronouns	-.08	-.24*	-.64
First person singular	.01	-.08	-.81#
Total first person	-.02	-.10	-.85*
Negations	-.03	.19#	.39
Assent	-.20*	-.26*	-.82*
Articles	.21*	.24*	.40
Prepositions	.20*	.19	-.36
Positive emotions	-.112	-.06	.75#
Anger	-.14#	-.20#	-.66
Cognitive processes	-.13	-.12	.73#
Discrepancies	.01	.05	.79#
Tentative	-.10	-.08	.78#
Friends	.02	.21#	.37
Family	.15‡	.18	.35
Past tense verbs	.16#	.08	.31
Present tense verbs	-.27***	-.16	.42
Space	-.14#	-.12#	-.64
Inclusive	.01	.01	.81#
School	.17*	.13	.45
Physical states	-.08	-.23#	-.64
Sleep	-.22**	-.26*	-.10
Swearing	-.14#	-.20#	-.66

*** two-tailed $p < .001$, ** two-tailed $p < .01$, * two-tailed $p < .05$, # trend (two-tailed $p < .10$)

19.1 Individual Posts

In the first analysis, the 145 posts were analyzed separately. As the postings got closer to Ashley's death, they increased in length and in the number of words per sentence. There was also a decrease in references to the present and a trend toward an increase in references to the past.

19.2 Posts by the Minute

In the second analysis, postings made within the same minute (for example, all postings made at 9:45) were combined into single texts, resulting in 75 texts to be compared. As with the first analysis, there was an increase in word count but, in this analysis, there was a decrease in words per sentence. There were trends toward a decrease in the use of anger words and an increase in references to friends.

19.3 Posts by the Hour

For the final analysis, postings made within the same hour (for example, all posts made between 10:00 am and 10:59 am) were combined. There was a trend toward a decrease in the use of the pronoun "I" and a significant decrease in references to the self. There was a trend toward an increase in positive emotion terms, but the decrease in negative emotions was not significant. The only finding that was statistically significant for all three analyses was that the use of assents (such as "yes" "ok" "mhmm") decreased over time.

19.4 Discussion

Several findings support the findings of previous research into written materials left behind by suicides. As with the study of Katie's diary (Chapter 3), there was an increase in positive emotions in the posts closer to death, but this finding was only a trend in the tweets. Also of interest was the decrease in references to the self.

The increase in positive emotions in the third analysis and the decrease in negative emotions, although they did not reach statistical significance, are consistent with the earlier studies of Katie's diary (Chapter 3) and the letters of a young man (Chapter 16). More importantly, they confirm clinical reports on patients residing on psychiatric wards who have been found, in retrospect, to show an improvement in mood in the hours prior to their suicide in the hospital.

A limitation of this analysis involves the nature of the postings. Each posting was relatively short and, when combined to be of an acceptable length (in the third analysis), there were only six postings for analysis. Finally, upon reading the posts, it becomes clear that Ashley attempted to write the posts using rhymes. For example: 10:21 am "I went to the bathroom and locked the door;" 10:22 am "I took apart a razor I had gotten from the store." As a result of her attempt to write poetically, Ashley may have used certain words that would not have been used if writing a suicide note or a journal entry. However, not all of the tweets rhymed in this way, and so this may be only a minor limitation.

As far as we can tell at the present time, Ashley came from a very dysfunctional family. She experienced accidents, bullying, sexual abuse, and a mother and stepfather who committed felonies. Her mother and grandmother had also been sexually abused in childhood which impaired their adult functioning. Ashley was a self-mutilator, had an eating disorder and psychiatric problems. In her tweets, of the ten warning signs posted on the website of the American Association of Suicidology,[72] six were present (suicidal ideation, purposelessness, anger, trapped, recklessness and mood change), indicating a high risk of suicide which clearly was indicated by her death from suicide hours later.

72 www.suicidology.org, with the mnemonic IS PATH WARM: suicidal ideation, substance abuse, purposelessness, anger, trapped, hopeless, withdrawal, anxiety, recklessness, and mood changes.

20 Interviews With Attempted Suicides

Turning Points (De Leo, 2010) presents us with moving written accounts from nine people who attempted to kill themselves, but who survived. All of them but one were happy to have survived. The question asked in this chapter is whether the essays written by these individuals provide clues to the suicidal mind.

20.1 The Attempters

20.1.1 Trevor

Trevor was a young man who became a drug and alcohol abuser. The woman he loved rejected him for another man, and his substance abuse worsened. He confided to no one. One night, he was drinking heavily and smoking dope, and he went home to change his clothes in order to go to a disco. He sat down and thought that he did not want to go out or do anything anymore. He got his roommate's shotgun and ammunition and waited for his friends to come by. He sat down and wrote a suicide note: *Tell Mum and Dad that I'm sorry and I love them.* He squeezed the trigger, but he had left the safety on. He tried again and, as he squeezed the trigger, changed his mind and tried to pull his head out of the way, but he shot much of the front of his head off.
De Leo noted that Trevor's account was rather "dry," and there is a lack of premeditation. There is also ambivalence as he waits for his friends to stop by. But Trevor seems to have little ability to self-monitor – to tell us what his mood and thoughts were.

20.1.2 Anna

Anna was sexually abused as a child by several men – neighbors, family friends and her grandfather. The abuse by her grandfather left her confused for she loved him and felt close to him but she knew what he was doing was wrong. He stopped abusing Anna when she was twelve, and he died two years later.

On the day that he died, Anna was stoic, "numb to the grief around me." She had been fighting with her parents to be allowed to go away with friends. Her relationship was "tumultuous" with her mother and distant with her step-father. Her brother and sister-in-law were "always there for me, but I felt such a burden on them." She felt hopeless and experienced despair. She went and got her grandfather's medications and ingested them all. "I am hopeless, bad at school, I can't get on with my parents, I am a burden to my support people, I cannot take another moment of this anguish. I can't cope anymore, I hate my life, I have nothing to live for" (p. 64).

Anna, therefore, illustrates common elements of the suicidal mind – psychological pain, hopelessness, and a sense of being a burden.

20.1.3 Alessa

Alessa was born into a wealthy family, but with a dysfunctional mother who could not cope with life and a father who was gone on business much of the time. Her mother made several suicide attempts with overdoses and, when Alessa was fifteen, she found her mother on the floor having tried to cut her throat. Alessa married, but her husband physically abused her and Alessa left him. Two months later she gave birth to a child with Down's syndrome. Alessa had a psychotic breakdown.

Alessa's mother changed dramatically at that time and became a good surrogate mother to her grandson, while Alessa continued to have symptoms of schizophrenia and became a drug addict. Eventually, Alessa recovered to some extent and got a job as a secretary when, one Easter, she decided it was time to die. "It happened all of a sudden....Basically, I wasn't doing badly. Yet that Saturday afternoon I decided that my hour had come, that the time was right, and that there was no point in going on' (p. 84). "I was suddenly overcome by the conviction that everything had been horrible and that I could no longer do anything with passion or hope. I was overcome by a sense of suffocating anxiety....My head was spinning and I felt I couldn't breathe anymore" (p. 85). She swallowed two laundry bottles of stain remover.
What is interesting here is the anxiety attack that immediately preceded her suicide attempt. She swallowed the poison in the midst of this emotion.

20.1.4 Sergio

Sergio, a father, felt responsible for letting his son drive a tractor when he was only twelve years old, which crashed and crippled the young boy. Sergio never recovered from the guilt, and his life became full of pain, guilt and a sense of oppression. In the months before his suicide attempt, this became unbearable. He could not sleep and began to drink heavily.

Sergio did not remember much of the day he tried to kill himself, but he remembered climbing the silo, shaking and crying. He thought that his pain would soon be over. But as soon as he jumped, he decided that he did not want to die. He reoriented himself while falling and damaged only his feet and ankles.

20.1.5 Sandro

Sandro became a concert pianist and married young. Although Sandro liked playing in bars, performing in concerts caused great tension for him. He began to drink, and eventually his wife left him. He was an alcoholic, with no job and no confidantes. He decided to kill himself.

He was sleeping only about two hours each night. He was tense and irritable, and yelling at his mother. One night at 2 am, he drove to his ex-wife's apartment and tried to kill himself with car exhaust. He wanted his ex-wife to see his corpse the next day. As he sat in the car, he drank some cognac and began writing a suicide note to his parents and to his ex-wife, mostly to her. He described the letter as full of accusations, anger, and threats.

20.1.6 Fabrizio

Fabrizio was diagnosed as having bipolar affective disorder at the age of 22. He lived in the countryside with his parents (his father was a policeman) and an uncle who shot himself at the age of 55. After his fourth or fifth admission for depression, Fabrizio began to think about suicide. During one hospitalization, Fabrizio met a woman whom he liked very much but who disappeared out of his life. During his last admission, he found out that she had hung herself. After his discharge he went home, got his father's gun and went into the basement. "I think my heart was beating fast. Rather strangely, while my head was in complete turmoil, my movements were correct and coordinated" (p. 115).

Again, like Alessa, Fabrizio reported only anxiety. Interestingly, he has two models for his choice – his uncle and the woman he liked – and he attempted suicide immediately after release from the psychiatric hospital, a common time for suicides in psychiatric patients.

20.1.7 Lucia

Lucia was married with two children. Her father, suffering from a bipolar disorder, killed himself using hanging when she was 27. His body was discovered by her younger brother. Her marriage was not good. There was no love and little sex. On the day, Lucia jumped from the third floor window of her apartment, she was tired from her work that day as a school teacher, and she reported a sensation of never-ending anxiety which she had been living with for some time.

Her husband, who was director of a museum, was tense that day and wanted Lucia to accompany him to a museum reception at which the Mayor was attending. There was tension between them in the car when she asked him to wait for her to go upstairs to the toilet. "I climbed the stairs again. It was suffocating inside there. My head was so heavy and my legs grew increasingly weaker.....I opened the door of the balcony....I didn't look down, I didn't hesitate – I just closed my eyes and I jumped....I thought that I was going to put an end to everything that was horrible and senseless. I was going to free myself, forever" (p. 124).

20.1.8 Umberto

Umberto was an old man and had to use a wheelchair. His wife had died of cancer fifteen years earlier, and his four children were grown up. His two daughters lived nearby but, "Even if I have cancer, I don't want my daughters to sacrifice their lives to remain close to me" (p. 130). Umberto spent time with a friend who had been crippled in a car wreck that killed his wife. Umberto secretly stole barbiturate pills from his friend over a period of months. He thought about using them to "reach" his wife whenever he chose to die, yet he did not believe in an afterlife. "What was there to live for?" He chose to overdose on the anniversary of his wife's death. He wrote notes to his children and to his friend. Worried that his friend would imitate him, Umberto wrote that, "my condition would have rapidly worsened anyway. More suffering, more medical visits, more interventions. More money spent, more assistance, more concern from my children. Better to end it as soon as possible" (p. 134). Umberto took the overdose and, in contrast to those above who reported being anxious in the moments leading up to the attempts, Umberto reported being calm.

20.1.9 Maria

Maria was an elderly lady, in a nursing home, who talked to Diego rather than writing. Maria suffered from a bipolar disorder and had attempted suicide in the past. Her life had been traumatic, with emigrations, the death of her husband and the suicides of her two sons. She jumped from the window of her apartment and suffered a spinal injury that left her paraplegic. "I don't know why I did it....and if someone would try to explain it to me, I would probably not believe it. The only thing that I remember is the tension that was devouring me, the incredible disquiet that I felt. I was confused. I could not clearly think about anything....I didn't want to suffer any more.....I did want to stop that tension, to put an end to that unbearable suffering. I am not sure if you really know what anxiety is, that particular anxiety. It is like a devil that bites you inside, that squeezes your lungs. You cannot breathe, you really cannot breathe" (pp. 147-148.).

20.2 Discussion

An interesting feature of these accounts is how little insight the people had into their mental state and their psychodynamics. They do illustrate several features well-known to suicidologists, such as escape from mental and physical pain (Sergio and Maria), anger (Sandro), hopelessness and a feeling of being a burden (Anna), and suicide soon after discharge from a psychiatric hospital (Fabrizio).

What is noteworthy is the anxiety noted by four of the individuals, Alessa, Fabrizio, Lucia and Maria. Alessa, Lucia and Maria all talk of suffocating and not being able to breathe any more, and two of them (Lucia and Maria) indicate that the anxiety was long-standing and not simply a result of the decision to kill themselves. In fact, Maria tried to die to get away from the anxiety. Anxiety has not been mentioned to any great extent in analyses of suicidal behavior. The focus has been on depression instead. These accounts indicate that clinicians should evaluate clients who are potentially suicidal for anxiety as well as depression and hopelessness.

Two other features also stand out. Four of the individuals had close relatives or friends who completed or attempted suicide, and it is well-known that having a significant other die from suicide is a risk factor for suicide. Second, five of the attempts were impulsive (Alessa, Fabrizio, Lucia, Maria and Trevor). Impulsive suicidal acts are very difficult for clinicians to predict and prevent.

21 Bereavement After Suicide: a Study of Memorials on the Internet[73]

When a person dies, those close to the deceased typically experience great sorrow, but the precise nature of the emotions experienced probably depends upon the cause of death. A death which is sudden and unexpected may have different consequences for the survivors than a death which was anticipated and for which the survivors had time to prepare. Even for unexpected deaths, the nature of the death may have an impact. Death from murder may leave survivors with different emotions than death from suicide or a heart attack. The other chapters in this book have attempted to understand the mind of the suicidal individual, but the present chapter explores the way in which the bereaved write about the suicide.

Death from suicide may result in a complex and intense set of emotional responses, including sadness, grief and anguish, as well as anger and guilt. Other emotions are aroused by the stigma that society attaches to suicide. The suicide of a person suggests the presence of psychiatric disorder in the deceased, and this leads to the suspicion that the whole family is psychiatrically disturbed. If the suicide was a respected and admired person in the community, friends may wonder what the relatives of the suicide did which drove the individual to take his own life.

To explore these issues, research into the aftermath of suicide has taken two separate approaches. The first strategy has been to ask the survivors of a suicide about their experiences, while the second strategy has been to ask members of the general public how they would view the survivors of a suicide. The first strategy focuses on the bereavement experience of the survivors of the suicide, while the second strategy focuses on the stigma that the survivors may have to face.

As Rudestam (1990) has pointed out, it is critically important to include an appropriate comparison group in studies of the bereaved survivors of a suicide. It is obvious that the survivors of a suicide will experience psychological and physical dysfunctions as part of the grief process. The crucial question, however, is whether these experiences differ from the grief process after a nonsuicidal death.

In addition, suicide may lead to reactions because the death was violent, guilt because the survivors feel they ought to have somehow intervened and prevented the suicide, and anger at the suicide for choosing to die in that particular manner. A suicidal death also has an effect on the mourning rituals, such as the funeral and religious services, and may lead to withdrawal of support from social networks because of the discomfort felt by neighbors and friends. Finally, the occurrence of a suicide suggests that the family system was dysfunctional already, and a dysfunctional

---

73 This chapter is based on Lester (2012).

family may have more difficulty in coming to terms with the death of a family member.

In a novel approach to this issue, Calhoun, Selby, and Steelman (1988-1989) asked funeral directors whether the mourners of a suicide differ from those of a natural death. Two main themes emerged. Family members of a suicide seemed to experience greater shock and more difficulty in dealing with the death, and the suicidal deaths seemed to generate more questioning in the mourners. The funeral directors themselves felt more constrained in dealing with the family of a suicide and had more difficulty in expressing sympathy and knowing what to say or do.

In studies of the emotional reactions of the bereaved, Rudestam (1977), for example, has documented relief, anger and depression in survivors of suicides, but research on those losing loved ones from other causes have shown that these emotions occur equally often in those individuals too (Calhoun, Selby, & Selby, 1982). The guilt experienced, however, does seem to be stronger in the survivors of a suicide (Glick, Weiss, & Parkes, 1974). Cognitive reactions in the survivors of suicide include shock and disbelief, a search for explanations, and denial. Studies which have included a comparison group have indicated that the search for explanations is more intense if the deceased was a suicide and less easily resolved (Sheskin & Wallace, 1976).

The circumstances of the suicide have been found to affect the resolution of these reactions. For example, Rudestam (1977) found that family members who discovered the body of the suicide were slower in recovering. The suicide can also make the resolution of grief difficult by the way he kills himself. For example, a person who shoots himself in the head, thereby disfiguring himself, in a locale where a loved one will discover his body, is clearly expressing anger toward the survivor. Discovering the deceased will be especially traumatic for the survivors.

Recent research continues to find differences in grief after a suicide versus other causes of death. For example, do Groot, de Keijser, and Neeleman (2006) found that survivors who had lost a relative to suicide, as compared to those who had lost a relative from natural causes, had higher scores on measures of neuroticism, loneliness, depression and complicated grief, lower scores on a measure of general health and expressed more a need for professional help three months after the death. Harwood, Hawton, Hope, and Jacoby (2002) found that survivors of suicide, as compared to survivors of natural deaths, felt more stigmatization, shame and a sense of rejection.

Mitchell, Kim, Prigerson, and Mortimer-Stephens (2004) found that survivors who lost a closely related person to suicide versus those who were only distantly related were significantly more likely to meet the criteria for complicated grief, a syndrome involving intrusive and distressing symptoms and symptoms of traumatization such as numbness, detachment and excessive anger and bitterness.

The present chapter takes a very different approach from previous research. Whereas previous research has administered questionnaires containing psychological and psychiatric inventories, the present study examined the memorials that survivors leave on Internet websites devoted to those grieving. Written memorials on a website for survivors of suicide were compared to those on a website for grief and loss in general using the LIWC.

All 17 memorials posted on the website www.spanusa.org were downloaded. Each was written by a suicide survivor, that is, someone who had lost a significant other to suicide. Fifteen were written by women and two by men. Nine had lost a child, four a sibling, two a spouse, one a parent, and one an employer. Seventeen comparison postings were obtained from www.grieflossrecovery.com. These were consecutive postings after eliminating postings that were about suicide (n = 2), not about death (n = 2), additional postings from the same person (n = 2), in a foreign language (n = 1), and about a dog (n = 1). The 34 postings were run through the LIWC program. Of the 73 comparisons, 13 were statistically significant and a further 13 tended toward statistical significance, many more than would be expected by chance in 73 statistical tests (see Table 21-1).

The postings from survivors of suicide had longer sentences and had a greater proportion of long words. They had fewer references to the deceased, more references to death, but fewer references to religion. They had more references to work, occupation, and school. They tended to have fewer references to the self, more references to anger and sadness, and fewer references to insight and understanding (words such as think, know, and consider).

Several significant differences had psychological relevance. For example, the memorials written by survivors of suicide had more references to death, had longer sentences and may be more complex as indicated by the use of more long words. The deaths from suicide, therefore, seemed to have a more profound impact on the survivors than the natural deaths. There were also more words reflecting anger and sadness, indicating more emotional distress, which is consistent with the research mentioned above which has found that complicated grief is more common to the survivors of suicide.

Finally, there were fewer words concerned with religion in the memorials written by survivors of suicide, suggesting that religion was less of a comfort for survivors of suicide than for survivors of natural deaths. Survivors of suicide are at increased risk of suicide themselves, perhaps because of inherited predispositions to psychiatric illness and the trauma of experience of the loss of a significant other to suicide (Runeson & Asberg, 2003), and it may be that conventional methods of alleviating the stress of loss, such as religion, are less effective for survivors of suicide.

Tab. 22.1: A comparison of written memorials from significant others who lost some to suicide versus other causes

	Grief website	Suicide website
Words per sentence	14.8	18.6**
Words longer than 6 letters	13.8	18.6***
Pronouns	15.9	13.1*
You	2.7	0.6*
Negations	2.0	1.1***
Senses	2.9	1.9**
Seeing	0.9	0.5*
Occupations	1.4	2.4**
School	0.3	0.8*
Job	0.3	0.7*
Religion	0.6	0.2*
Death	0.7	1.3*
Eating	0.3	0.1*
Words in the dictionary	80.4	77.7#
First person singular	6.3	4.6#
Total first person	8.0	6.2#
Prepositions	12.5	13.7#
Anger	0.2	0.4#
Sad	1.0	1.4#
Insight	2.3	1.9#
Inhibition	0.3	0.5#
Hearing	1.2	0.8#
Friends	0.2	0.3#
Humans	0.6	0.9#
Time	5.6	4.8#
Music	0.15	0.04#

*** two-tailed $p < .001$, ** two-tailed $p < .01$, * two-tailed $p < .05$, # trend (two-tailed $p < .10$)

22 Conclusions: What Have We Learned?

This book has presented both qualitative and quantitative analyses of the writings left by suicides in their diaries, suicide notes, poems, letters, twitter feeds, blogs and tape recordings. My first reaction was how powerful the diaries that I have read are, and this is especially true for the diaries that I was given by those bereaved by the suicide of a loved one. The writers of those diaries present in clear, emotional and moving words the conflicts that they are experiencing. Compared to these diaries, suicide notes are very brief and often fail to provide any clues to what was in the minds of those about to kill themselves. The diaries provide scores, even hundreds, of pages describing the writer's pain.

Let me review my thoughts on this project.

22.1 Biographies versus Diaries

I started this project in order to satisfy myself. If my research, and the research of others, fails to provide an insight into the mind of the suicidal individual, might the study of their diaries provide this insight? I had read biographies of famous individuals who had taken their own lives, and these provide some clues about the life paths that end in some people killing themselves. But biographies are written by an outsider, someone who knows the facts about, but not the mind of, the protagonist. The diaries give us a window into their mind.

The facts of a person's life are, of course, important, but combining the facts with the words of the protagonist is immeasurably better. For example, the biography of Cesare Pavese by Lajolo (1983) (discussed in Chapter 4) is important in framing the life of Pavese. Pavese's novels, which reflect his personal life, also provide insight into his mind. But his diary, despite the translation and possible editing, gives us insight into his thought processes which illuminate the facts of his life, information which is not present in Lajolo's biography of Pavese or in Pavese's own novels.

Of course, for the personal diaries given to me by the significant others of those who died by suicide, there is no biography. In my analysis of the letters written by Clara (Chapter 16), a biography of her life would have provided better insights into the psychodynamics motivating her choice of suicide. But no detailed biographies are available for the writers of these private diaries, only the sketchy outline of their life paths.

The published diaries (such as that from Cesare Pavese) are typically accompanied by extensive biographies, but these diaries may have been written by those who knew that their diaries would eventually be published. Thus, they may have been edited by the writer, in addition to edits made by the scholar who presented them for publication. Thus, they are likely to be more constrained and more intellectual in tone.

22.2 Qualitative versus Quantitative Methodologies

The chapters in this book have used both clinical insight and quantitative analysis. My clinical analysis of the diary of the university professor (Robert in Chapter 7) provides a detailed description of the conflicts and psychological pain that Robert was experiencing, and it is surprising to me that he lived as long as he did. For some of the diaries, it was possible also to run the text through the LIWC program. Sometimes, this confirmed the clinical insights, as when it clearly identified the increase in positive emotions and the decrease in negative emotions over time in Katie's diary (Chapter 3), which was noted impressionistically by Silvia Canetto (2004) in her chapter in my book *Katie's Diary* (Lester, 2004b). On occasions, the LIWC identified trends that a simple reading of the diaries would not identify. For example, the increase in question marks in Katie's diary identified by the LIWC program (Pennebaker & Stone, 2004) is intriguing even if we, as yet, can provide no interpretation for this trend.

There is often a conflict between those engaged in, and advocating, the two methodologies. In particular, those who produce qualitative studies often feel that their contributions have greater difficulty getting published and, when published, are often ignored.[74] Antoon Leenaars and his colleagues edited a special issue of the *Archives of Suicide Research* (2002, volume 6, number 1) in which this conflict was discussed, with proponents of qualitative methodologies (e.g., Gerisch, 2002) and proponents of quantitative methodologies (e.g., de Wilde, 2002) both represented. I argued that the two methodologies could complement each other (Lester, 2002b). For example, Clarke and Lester (2013) showed that the choice of method for suicide is affected greatly by the ease of obtaining the means (such as toxic domestic gas) for that method. On the other hand, case studies, a qualitative method, can indicate why *this person* chose *that method*. For example, Grumet (1989), commenting on a male nurse who used an overdose and an electrocution to attempt suicide, noted that the use of electrocution was motivated symbolically by a desire to cure himself of his psychiatric disorder (he had wanted to have electroconvulsive therapy) and as a wish to be punished for being bad (an execution by electrocution).

The analyses in this book, therefore, illustrate the ways in which qualitative and quantitative approaches can complement each other rather than being rival methodologies. Indeed, the analysis of Jim's diary (Chapter 6) used a qualitative analysis of themes, the results from the LIWC computer program, and insights from Jim's sister, providing three different but complementary views of Jim's life.

---

74 These two approaches parallel to some extent the age-old distinction between idiographic approach (the study of the individual) and the nomothetic approach (the study of samples of individuals).

22.3 Poems and Letters

The study of the poems written by those who died by suicide provided fewer clues into the mind of the writer, probably because poems are crafted carefully by the writer, whereas diaries are rarely changed and edited by their writers. Even though Arthur Inman (Chapter 5) could have edited his diary when his assistants typed the pages, he steadfastly refused to change a word. He wanted his diary to be exactly as he wrote it, even if he changed his mind about what he had written and even if the words insulted or hurt those around him who were typing it. Even Katie's poems (Chapter 15), which not written by an accomplished poet and not intended for publication, gave little insight into the conflicts behind her choice of suicide.

The study of letters (Chapter 16) was also somewhat disappointing. Those of van Gogh revealed little personal information, and those of Clara were written many months before her death by suicide and seemed to be quite superficial in tone. The letters of the young man to a close friend (to whom he was probably attracted) showed some trends consistent with the findings from the studies of the diaries, such as the changes in positive and negative emotions, but the content of the letters gave few clues to his conflicts and his mental pain. Since letters are written for others to read, perhaps the writers are more constrained in what they put down on paper (or write in an e-mail).

Suicide notes are written in the minutes (or hours) prior to death and are less likely to be edited and constrained by the formalities of writing that are present in letters and poems. This is not to argue that we should not study such letters and poems. Those who die by suicide leave so little behind for us to explore the psychodynamics of their choice of suicide that we must use whatever we can find. Occasionally, too, we find a wonderful poem or letter that throws light on the person's choice. For example, Sylvia Plath's poem *Daddy* (Plath, 1981; see Chapter 1 above) provides clues to her choice of suicide.

The analysis of tweets (Chapter 19) and tape recordings (Chapter 18) also provide uncensored and unedited words from people in the period just before they died by suicide. De Leo's interviews with survivors of suicide attempts (Chapter 21) presented the unedited words of people, and de Leo's sensitive interviewing identified psychological processes that have not been mentioned much in the past (such as the role of anxiety in the moments prior to the suicidal action).

22.4 Suicide Notes

Suicide notes have been studied using judges to rate the presence of general themes in many prior studies. For example, Leenaars, et al. (1992b) rated suicide notes for the presence of Karl Menninger's three major themes (anger-in, anger-out, and escape), and Gunn, et al. (2012) rated the presence of the themes from Joiner's (2005) theory of suicide (thwarted belonging and perceived burdensomeness). Such studies are often impaired by poor agreement between the raters, and the use of the LIWC program avoids these inconsistencies.

The noteworthy finding of the analyses in Part 2 of this book has been the difference in the results when a large sample of suicide notes is available. In the past, researchers have been constrained by the small samples that they have been able to collect, typically forty or so suicide notes at most. The analysis of the 260 notes from Australia provided much richer results. For example, whereas previous research had identified few, if any, differences in the content of suicide notes written by men and by women, the present analysis in Chapter 13 of the sample of 260 suicide notes identified many differences. The suicide notes written by women referred more to themselves, and contained more positive emotions and references to thought processes and insight (perhaps because they gave more reasons for their choice of suicide).

As noted in Chapter 11, the study of suicide notes was, in my opinion, hindered by the publication by Shneidman and Farberow (1957b) of 33 pairs of genuine and simulated suicide notes. Because of the difficulties of obtaining samples of suicide notes, researchers used these notes for some two dozen studies. I argued that these studies do not throw much light on the suicidal mind but, rather, on lay theories of suicides – what nonsuicidal people think is going on in the mind of the suicidal person. The ideal comparison group should not be simulated suicide notes written by nonsuicidal people, but instead letters and notes written by the suicides a year or more earlier. No researcher has ever attempted to collect such a comparison sample of notes. However, diaries do accomplish this. The last entry prior to the death can be compared with an entry one year earlier. The drawback, of course, is that the sample size is tiny. Part 1 of this book discussed only eight diaries of suicides (if we include Bobby Sands), and I have only recently acquired a ninth diary.

22.5 “Firsts”

The present book contained many “firsts.”

(1) The study of eight diaries is the first major study of diaries. Lester (2004) provided the first study of one diary, but this book begins the project of collecting a sample of diaries so that we can distinguish general themes from idiosyncratic themes. The inclusion of a diary from a hunger-striker (Bobby Sands in Chapter 10), which showed no resemblance to any of the other diaries, indicated that the diaries of those who die by suicide may have unique properties.

(2) The study of Twitter postings by a young girl written in the hours before her death by suicide (see Chapter 19) illustrated the possibilities that modern media outlets provide for studies of what is transpiring in the mind of the suicide prior to the act. The study of these types of material may be affected by the fact that the individuals know that their Tweets, YouTube video or Facebook posting will be viewed by

others and, therefore, will be affected by the image that the potential suicides wish to convey but this is true for suicide notes also. Yang and Lester (2011) argued that we should not always believe the truthfulness of the content in suicide notes since writers of such notes are often trying to shape their image so that they are remembered in a particular way by their significant others.

(3) The study of the two tape recordings made the young man in the hours before he died by suicide (Chapter 18) provide the first ever insight into the mind of potential suicides immediately prior to their deaths. As I noted in Chapter 18 (and throughout the book), two research teams had reported that the mood of the suicide seemed to improve in the hours prior to their death, and this was clearly documented in the two tapes left by the young man. The second recording was calmer and more other-oriented than the first tape.

(4) The discussion of Diego de Leo's (2010) book (Chapter 21) reporting his interviews with those who made serious attempts to die by suicide, but who failed, shows how little insight that individuals have into their own minds. The more formal analysis of the written and spoken words of suicidal individuals provides much more information. However, as I noted in Chapter 21, where I reviewed the accounts of these attempted suicides, the role of anxiety in the minutes prior to their suicidal act came through clearly in their accounts, and this had not been identified by the more formal research conducted on attempted suicides in the hours and days after their actions using standardized psychological tests.

22.6 Understanding the Mind of the Suicidal Individual

Although those who are suicidal or about to attempt or complete suicide can tell us what the precipitating event is, they are often unaware of the psychodynamics behind their act. In scholarly terms, they can tell us about the stress but not the diathesis. Even the most popular theory of suicide in recent years, that proposed by Joiner (2005), can tell us only about the triggering events (thwarted belongingness and perceived burdensomeness), but nothing about why some people react to a thwarted relationship by killing themselves while most do not. These theories of suicide also tell us very little about what is going on in the mind of the suicidal person. We should note in passing that, even when suicidal individuals do have some insight, as in the case of Sylvia Plath, this does not prevent their suicide.

The words of the suicides, written or spoken, clearly attest to the immense psychological distress in their minds. There is a world of difference between a word like Shneidman's (1996) *psychache* and the expression of this pain in Katie's diary (Chapter 3) or Stephen's spoken words (Chapter 18). For some of the people discussed in this book, this pain seems to lessen in the hours (Stephen) or days and weeks (Katie) before the suicide but, prior to that, the pain is raw.

It does appear that we have underestimated the role of anxiety in the moments prior to a suicide. De Leo's interviews with survivors of attempted suicide documented this anxiety, but so does the diary of Arthur Inman (Chapter 5). Although the published diary omits the entries from the final few months, I have perused the handwritten entries for the final month and can attest to the presence of acute anxiety in Inman in the days before he killed himself.

The existence of schemata in which one thought leads to another and then another wa proposed by Kovacs and Beck (1978), and this was evident in the diaries of Cesare Pavese (Chapter 4) and Robert (Chapter 7). In Pavese's case, failure in love led to thoughts that he was a failure as a writer. In Robert's case, anxiety over his teaching and scholarly work led to thoughts of his Oedipal complex and sexual conflicts. In addition, in Robert's case, the way in which one pejorative word about himself led to a seemingly well-rehearsed sequence of such words was noteworthy.

Cognitive theories of suicide have often noted the tunnel vision (cognitive constriction) and rigidity in the thinking of suicidal people. This was evident, for example, in the diary of Inman who saw no alternative to his living situation. Either he had to stay where he was living, or he had to kill himself. However, it is interesting to see how Jim (Chapter 6) also constructed the situation so that he had no other choice. He killed himself when he ran out of money. His electricity was about to be cut off, his house would be seized, and he had no money left for food or alcohol – not one cent. Jim constructed the cost-benefit analysis of the decision to die by suicide so that the benefit outweighed the cost.

It is important to note that the suicides discussed in this book are more dissimilar from one another than similar. Although it is possible to draw some parallels, they are very different. Katie has romantic relationship problems, but Pavese has no romantic relationships (only fantasies). Inman cannot tolerate situational change (moving house), while Robert cannot tolerate a negative academic judgment (a failure to obtain tenure). Inman is anxious, but Jim is resigned.

Even when there are similarities, there are slight differences. Pavese's diary showed an increase in positive emotions over the last few months of the diary but, in the letters from a young man to his friend (Chapter 16), there was a decrease in negative emotions. The overall mood in both improved, but for different reasons. There are, therefore, perhaps no generalizations we can draw about every suicide. Not surprisingly, each is unique.

Finally, it is interesting to note that theories of suicide have little to say about the suicides presented and discussed in this book. Instead, the classic theories of personality (such as psychoanalytic theory) and the classic systems of psychotherapy (such as cognitive therapy) provide a better framework for analyzing and understanding these suicides.

22.7 Final Thoughts

The present book has shown the importance of "listening" to the words that those about to die by suicide say and write. Our formal psychological tests provide useful information and enable us to test our theories of suicide, but they fail to capture the pain and the thought processes of the suicidal person. Biographies of suicides and clinical reports of cases are, of course, interesting, but they are far removed from the experiences of the protagonists. Only their own words can give us clues as to what is transpiring in the "I" of the storm.

References

Aaron, D. (1985). *The Inman diary: A public and private confession*. Cambridge, MA: Harvard University Press.

Agnew, R. (1992). Foundations for a general strain theory. *Criminology*, 30, 47-88.

Allport, G. (1942). *The use of personal documents in psychological science*. New York: Social Science Research Council.

Allport, G. W. (1965). *Letters from Jenny*. New York: Harcourt, Brace & World.

Andreasen, N. C. (1987). Creativity and mental illness. *American Journal of Psychiatry*, 144, 1288-1292.

Angyal, A. (1965). *Neurosis and treatment*. New York: Wiley.

Ansbacher, H. L. (1961). Suicide. In N. L. Farberow & E. S. Shneidman (Eds.) *The cry for help*, pp. 204-219. New York: McGraw-Hill.

Baker, W. E. (1913) Diary of a suicide. *The Glebe*, 1(2), 7-83.

Balance, W. D., & Leenaars, A. A. (1986). A predictive approach to Aaron Beck's formulations regarding suicide. In R. Cohen-Sandler (Ed.) *Proceedings of the 19th Annual Meeting*, p. 51. Denver, CO: American Association of Suicidology.

Bantum, E. O., & Owen, J. E. (2009). Evaluating the validity of computerized content analysis programs for identification of emotional expression in cancer narratives. *Psychological Assessment*, 21, 79-88.

Barnes, D. H., Lawal-Solarin, F. W., & Lester, D. (2007). Letters from a suicide. *Death Studies*, 31, 671-678.

Baumeister, R. F. (1990). Suicide as escape from self. *Psychological Review*, 97, 90-113.

Beck, A. T. (1991). Cognitive therapy. *American Psychologist*, 46, 368-375.

Beck, J. S. (1996). Cognitive therapy of personality disorders. In P. M. Salkovskis (Ed.) *Frontiers of cognitive therapy*, pp. 165-181. New York: Guilford.

Binswanger, L. (1958). The case of Ellen West. In R. May, E. Angel & H. F. Ellenberger (Eds.) *Existence*, pp. 237-364. New York: Basic Books.

Black, S. T. (1989). Gender differences in the content of genuine and simulated suicide note. In D. Lester (Ed.) *Suicide '89*, p. 8. Denver, CO: American Association of Suicidology.

Black, S. T. (1993). Comparing genuine and simulated suicide notes. *Journal of Consulting & Clinical Psychology*, 61, 699-702.

Black, S. T., & Lester, D. (1995). Distinguishing suicide notes from completed suicides and attempted suicides. *Perceptual & Motor Skills*, 81, 802.

Black, S. T., & Lester, D. (2001). The use of substitute subjects in the study of suicide. *European Journal of Psychiatry*, 15, 133-136.

Bond, G. D., & Lee, A. Y. (2005). Language of lies in prison. *Applied Cognitive Psychology*, 19, 313-329.

Brevard, A., & Lester, D. (1991). A comparison of suicide notes written by completed and attempted suicides. *Annals of Clinical Psychiatry*, 3, 43-45.

Brevard, A., Lester, D., & Yang, B. (1990). A comparison of suicide notes written by suicide completers and suicide attempters. *Crisis*, 11, 7-11.

Brumberg, J. J. (1997). *The body project*. New York: Random House.

Calhoun, L, G., Selby, J. W., & Selby, L. E. (1982). The psychological aftermath of suicide. *Clinical Psychology Review, 2*, 409-420.

Calhoun, L. G., Selby, J. W., & Steelman, J. (1988-1989). A collation of funeral directors' impressions of suicidal deaths. *Omega, 19*, 365-373.

Canetto, S. S. (1992-1993). She died for love and he for glory. *Omega*, 26, 1-17.

Canetto, S. S. (2004). Why did you kill yourself, Katie? In D. Lester (Ed.) *Katie's diary,* pp.41-54. New York: Brunner-Routledge.
Canetto, S. S., & Lester, D. (Eds.) (1995). *Women and suicidal behavior.* New York: Springer.
Cavan, R. S. (1965). *Suicide.* New York: Russell & Russell.
Clarke, J., & van Amerom, G. (2008). A comparison of blogs by depressed men and women. *Issues in Mental Health Nursing*, 29, 243-264.
Clarke, R. V., & Lester, D. (2013). *Suicide: Closing the exits.* New Brunswick, NJ: Transaction.
Clements, C., Bonacci, D., Yerevanian, B., Privitera, M., & Kiehne, L. (1985). Assessment of suicide risk in patients with personality disorder and major affective disorder. *Quality Review Bulletin*, 11(5), 150-154.
Culley, M. (1985). *A day at a time.* New York: Feminist Press at CUNY.
Dabrowski, K. (1964). *Positive disintegration.* Boston, MA: Little Brown.
Darbonne, A. R. (1967). An investigation into the communication style of suicidal individuals. *Dissertation Abstracts*, 27B, 2504-2505.
Davies, R. (1993). *The Kenneth Williams diaries.* London, UK: HarperCollins.
De Catanzaro, D. (1980). *Suicide and self-damaging behavior.* New York: Academic.
de Groot, M. H., de Keijser, J., & Neeleman, J. (2006). Grief shortly after suicide and natural death. *Suicide & Life-Threatening Behavior, 36,* 418-431.
De Leo, D. (2010). *Turning points.* Bowen Hills, Australia: Australian Academic Press.
de Wilde, E. J. (2002). Quantitative research in suicidology. *Archives of Suicide Research, 6,* 55-59.
Djikic, M., & Oatley, K. (2006). The bitter-sweet labor of emoting. *Creativity Research Journal*, 18, 191-197.
Dollard, J., & Mowrer, O. H. (1947). A method of measuring tension in written documents. *Journal of Abnormal & Social Psychology*, 42, 3-32.
Drake, W. (1979). *Sara Teasdale.* New York: Harper & Row.
Durkheim, E. (1897). *Le suicide.* Paris, France: Felix Alcan.
Edelman, A., & Renshaw, S. (1982). Genuine versus simulated suicide notes. *Suicide & Life-Threatening Behavior*, 12, 103-113.
Ellis, T. E. (2004). Thoughts of Katie. In D. Lester (Ed.) *Katie's diary*, pp. 81-96. New York: Brunner-Routledge.
Everson, L. (2006). *Everything preserved.* Saint Paul, MN: Graywolf Press.
Faber, M. (1970). *Suicide and Greek tragedy.* New York: Sphinx Press.
Frankl, V. E. (1963). *Man's search for meaning.* New York: Pocket Books.
Frederick, C. J. (1968). An investigation of handwriting of suicidal persons through suicide notes. *Journal of Abnormal Psychology*, 73, 263-267.
Gerisch, B. (2002). Aspects of qualitative research in suicidology. *Archives of Suicide Research, 6,* 31-39.
Glick, I. O., Weiss, R. S., & Parkes, M. P. (1974). *The first year of bereavement.* New York: Wiley.
Goodwin, D. W. (1988). *Alcohol and the writer.* Kansas City, MO: Andrews & McMeel.
Gottschalk, L. A., & Gleser, G. C. (1960). An analysis of the verbal content of suicide notes. *British Journal of Medical Psychology*, 33, 195-204.
Grumet, G. W. (1989). Attempted suicide by electrocution. *Bulletin of the Menninger Clinic, 53,* 512-521.
Gunn, J. F., & Lester, D. (2012). Twitter postings and suicide. *Suicidologi,* 17(3), 28-30.
Gunn, J. F., Lester, D., Haines, J., & Williams, C. L. (2012). Thwarted belongingness and perceived burdensomeness in suicide notes. *Crisis*, 33, 178-181.
Gut, E. (1989). *Productive and unproductive depression.* New York: Basic Books.
Haines, J., Williams, C. L., & Lester, D. (2010). Completed suicides: Is there method in their madness? *Clinical Neuropsychiatry*, 7, 133-140.

Handelman, L. D., & Lester, D. (2007). The content of suicide notes from attempters and completers. *Crisis*, 28, 102-104.

Harwood, D., Hawton, K., Hope, T., & Jacoby, R. (2002). The grief experiences and needs of bereaved relatives and friends of older people dying through suicide. *Journal of Affective Disorders*, 72, 185-194.

Hendin, H. (1964). *Suicide in Scandinavia*. New York: Grune & Stratton.

Henken, V. (1976). Banality revisited. *Suicide & Life-Threatening Behavior*, 6, 36-43.

Hirsh, J. B., & Peterson, J. B. (2009). Personality and language use in self-narratives. *Journal of Research in Personality*, 43, 524-527.

Holden, C. (1987). Creativity and the troubled mind. *Psychology Today*, 21(4), 9-10.

Hookway, N. (2008). Entering the blogosphere. *Qualitative Research*, 8, 91-113.

Huffaker, D. A., & Calvert, S. L. (2005). Gender, identity, and language use in teenage blogs. *Journal of Computer-Mediated Communication*, 10(2), online.

Inman, A. C. (1985). *The Inman diary*. Ed. by D. Aaron. Cambridge, MA: Harvard University Press.

Jacobs, J. (1967). A phenomenological study of suicide notes. *Social Problems*, 15, 60-72.

Jaffe, A. (1967). *The process of Kafka's trial*. East Lansing, MI: Michigan State University Press.

Jang, S. H. (2004). Continuing suicide among laborers. *Labor History*, 45, 271-297.

Janson, M. P., Alessandrini, E. S., Strunjas, S. S., Shahab, H., El-Mallakh, R., & Lippmann, S. b. (2001). Internet-observed suicide attempts. *Journal of Clinical Psychiatry*, 62, 478.

Jardine, L. (1983). *Still harping on daughters*. Totowa, NJ: Barnes & Noble.

Johnson, B. D. (1965). Durkheim's one cause of suicide. *American Sociological Review*, 30, 875-886.

Joiner, T. (2005). *Why people die by suicide*. Cambridge, MA: Harvard University Press.

Joiner, T. E., Pettit, J. W., Walker, R. L., Voelz, Z. R., Cruz, J., Rudd, M. D., & Lester, D. (2002). Perceived burdensomeness and suicidality. *Journal of Social & Clinical Psychology*, 21, 531-545.

Jourard, S. (1971). *Self-disclosure*. New York: Wiley.

Junghaenel, D., Smyth, J. M., & Santner, L. (2008). Linguistic dimensions of psychopathology. *Journal of Social & Clinical Psychology*, 27, 36-55.

Justice, D. (Ed.) (2003). *The collected poems of Weldon Kees*. Lincoln, NE: University of Nebraska Press.

Kagle, S. E. (1979). *American diary literature, 1620-1799*. Boston, MA: Twayne.

Keith-Spiegel, P., & Spiegel, D. E. (1967). Affective states of patients immediately preceding suicide. *Journal of Psychiatric Research*, 5, 89-93.

Kelly, G. A. (1955). *The psychology of personal constructs*. New York: Norton.

Kim, Y. S. (2008). Bullying and suicide: a review. *International Journal of Adolescent Medicine & Health*, 20, 133-154.

Klest, B., & Freyd, J. (2007). Global ratings of essays about trauma. *Journal of Psychological Trauma*, 6(1), 1-20.

Kovacs, M., & Beck, A. T. (1978). Maladaptive cognitive structures in depression. *American Journal of Psychiatry*, 135, 525-533.

Kramer, D. A. (2002). A psychobiographical analysis of faith, hope, and despair in suicide. *Journal of Adult Development*, 9, 117-126.

Laing, R. D. (1960). *The divided self*. London, UK: Tavistock.

Lajolo, D. (1983). *An absurd vice*. New York: New Directions.

Lee, C. H., Park, J., & Seo, J. (2006). An analysis of linguistic styles by inferred age in TV dramas. *Psychological Reports*, 99, 351-356.

Leenaars, A. A. (1988a). *Suicide notes*. New York: Human Sciences Press.

Leenaars, A. A. (1988b) Are women's suicides really different from men's? *Women & Health*, 18, 17-33.

Leenaars, A. A. (1989). Suicide across the adult life-span. *Crisis*, 10, 132-151.

Leenaars, A. A., & Lester, D. (1991). Myths about suicide notes. *Death Studies*, 15, 303-308.

Leenaars, A. A., Lester, D., Wenckstern, S., McMullin, C., Rudzinski, D., & Brevard, A. (1992a). Comparison of suicide notes and parasuicide notes. *Death Studies*, 16, 331-342.
Leenaars, A. A., Lester, D., & Yang, B. (1992b). Menninger's motives for suicide in the notes of completed and attempted suicides. *Psychological Reports*, 70, 369-370.
Leenaars, A. A., & Maltsberger, J. T. (1994). The Inman diary. In A. A. Leenaars, J. T. Maltsberger & R. A. Neimeyer (Eds.) *Treatment of suicidal people*, pp. 227-236. Washington, DC: Taylor & Francis.
Leenaars, A. A., McLister, D., & Balance, W. (1989).An empirical investigation of the latent content of suicide notes. In D. Lester (Ed.) *Suicide '89*, pp. 282-283. Denver, CO: American Association of Suicidology.
Lepore, S. J., & Smyth, J. M. (2002). *The writing cure*. Washington, DC: American Psychological Association.
Lester, D. (1969). Resentment and dependency in the suicidal individual. *Journal of General Psychology*, 81, 137-145.
Lester, D. (1971a). Ellen West's suicide as a case of psychic homicide. *Psychoanalytic Review*, 58, 251-263.
Lester, D. (1971b). Need for affiliation in suicide notes. *Perceptual & Motor Skills*, 33, 550.
Lester, D. (1971c). Need for affiliation in suicide notes. *Perceptual & Motor Skills*, 33, 550.
Lester, D. (1971d). Choice of method for suicide and personality. *Omega*, 2, 76-80.
Lester, D. (1972). Suicide in Ibsen's plays. *Life-Threatening Behavior*, 2, 35-41.
Lester, D. (1973). Temporal perspective and completed suicide. *Perceptual & Motor Skills*, 36, 760.
Lester, D. (1984). Suicide. In C. S. Widom (Ed.) *Sex roles and psychopathology.*, pp. 145-156. New York: Plenum.
Lester, D. (1987). Psychology and literature. *Psychology*, 24(1/2), 25-27.
Lester, D. (1988a). What does the study of simulated suicide notes tell us? *Psychological Reports*, 62, 962.
Lester, D. (1988b). Excitor-inhibitor scales of the MMPI and choice of method for suicide. *Perceptual & Motor Skills*, 66, 218.
Lester, D. (1989a). Application of Piotrowski's dark shading hypothesis to Sylvia Plath's poems written before her suicide. *Perceptual & Motor Skills*, 68, 122.
Lester, D. (1989b). Experience of parental loss and later suicide. *Acta Psychiatrica Scandinavica*, 79, 450-452.
Lester, D. (1989c). Menninger's motives for suicide in genuine and simulated suicide notes. *Perceptual & Motor Skills*, 69, 850.
Lester, D. (1991a). Reliability of naive judges of genuine suicide notes. *Perceptual & Motor Skills*, 73, 942.
Lester, D. (1991b). Accuracy of recognition of genuine versus simulated suicide. *Personality & Individual Differences*, 12, 765-766.
Lester, D. (1991c). Dark-shading in the poems of Anne Sexton. *Perceptual & Motor Skills*, 73, 366.
Lester, D. (1993). Reliability of judging genuine and simulated suicide notes. *Perceptual & Motor Sills*, 77, 882.
Lester, D. (1994a). Motives for suicide in suicide notes from completed and attempted suicides. *Psychological Reports*, 75, 1130.
Lester, D. (1994b). Can suicidologists distinguish between suicide notes from completers and attempters? *Perceptual & Motor Skills*, 79, 1498.
Lester, D. (1994c). Correlates of accuracy in judging genuine versus simulated suicide notes. *Perceptual & Motor Skills*, 79, 642.
Lester, D. (1995a). Personality correlates of correctly identifying genuine suicide notes. *Perceptual & Motor Skills*, 80, 890.
Lester, D. (1995b). *Theories of personality*. Philadelphia, PA: Taylor & Francis.
Lester, D. (2002a). The scientific study of suicide requires accurate data. *Crisis*, 23, 133-134.

Lester, D. (2002b). Qualitative versus quantitative studies in psychiatry. *Archives of Suicide Research, 6,* 15-18.
Lester, D. (2004a). The Ophelia complex. In D. Lester (Ed.) *Katie's diary*, pp. 109-122. New York: Brunner-Routledge.
Lester, D. (Ed.). (2004b). *Katie's dairy.* New York: Brunner-Routledge.
Lester, D. (2006). Understanding suicide through studies of diaries: the case of Cesare Pavese. *Archives of Suicide Research*, 10, 295-302.
Lester, D. (2009). Learning about suicide from the diary of Cesare Pavese. *Crisis*, 30, 222-224.
Lesterd, D. (2010a) *A multiople self theory of personality*. Hauppauge, NY: Nova Science.
Lester, D. (2010b). The reasons for suicide: an analysis of the diary of Arthur Inman. *Death Studies*, 34, 54-70.
Lester, D. (2010c). Linguistic analysis of a blog from a murder-suicide. *Psychological Reports*, 106, 342.
Lester, D. (2010d). The final hours. *Psychological Reports*, 106, 791-797.
Lester, D. (2012). Bereavement and suicide. *Omega,* 65, 189-194.
Lester, D., & Beck, A. T. (1980-1981). What the suicide's choice of method signifies. *Omega,* 11, 271-277.
Lester, D., & Heim, N. (1992). Sex differences in suicide notes. *Perceptual & Motor Skills*, 75, 582.
Lester, D. & Hummel, H. (1980). Motives for suicide in elderly people. *Psychological Reports*, 47, 870.
Lester, D., & Leenaars, A. A. (1987). Differentiation of genuine suicide notes. *Psychological Reports*, 61, 70.
Lester, D., & Leenaars, A. A. (1988). The moral justification of suicide in suicide notes. *Psychological Reports*, 63, 106.
Lester, D., & Linn, M. (1997). Sex differences in suicide notes. *Psychological Reports*, 80, 1302.
Lester, D., & Reeve, C. (1982). The suicide notes of young and old people. *Psychological Reports*, 50, 334.
Lester, D., Seiden, R. H., & Tauber, R. K. (1990). Menninger's motives for suicide in genuine, simulated and hoax suicide notes. *Perceptual & Motor Skills*, 71, 248.
Lester, D., & Terry, R. (1992). The use of poetry therapy. *The Arts in Psychotherapy*, 19, 47-52.
Lester, D., & Terry, R. (1993-1994). Emotional self-repair and poetry. *Omega*, 28, 79-84.
Linn, M., & Lester, D. (1996). Content differences in suicide notes by gender and age. *Psychological Reports*, 78, 370.
Livermore, A. (1985). Forty suicide notes. In R. Cohen-Sandler (Ed.) *Proceedings of the 18th Annual Meeting*, pp. 47-49. Denver, CO: American Association of Suicidology.
McGee, A. (1987). *The Elizabethan Hamlet*. New Haven, CT: Yale University Press.
McLister, B., & Leenaars, A. A. (1988). An empirical investigation of the latent content of suicide notes. *Psychological Reports*, 63, 238.
Meerloo, J. A. M. (1962). *Suicide and mass suicide*. New York: Grune & Stratton.
Meyer, M. (1971). *Ibsen*. New York: Doubleday.
Mitchell, A. M., Kim, Y., Prigerson, H. G., & Mortimer Stephens, M. (2004). Complicated grief in survivors of suicide. *Crisis,* 25, 12-18.
Mosak, H., & Maniacci, M. (1999). *A primer of Adlerian psychology*. Philadelphia, PA: Brunner-Routledge.
Musto, D. F. (1985). A medical report on Arthur Inman. In. D. Aaron (Ed.) *The Inman diary: A public and private confession*, pp. 1603-1618. Cambridge, MA: Harvard University Press.
Neuringer, C. (1988). The thinking processes in suicidal women. In D. Lester (Ed.) *Why women kill themselves*, pp. 43-52. Springfield, IL: Charles C. Thomas.
Neuringer, C., & Lettieri, D. J. (1982). *Suicidal women*. New York: Gardner.

Nolen-Hoeksema, S. (1987). Sex differences in unipolar depression. *Psychological Bulletin*, 101, 259-282.

Nolen-Hoeksema, S., Larson, J., & Grayson, C. (1999). Explaining the gender difference in depressive symptoms. *Journal of Personality & Social Psychology*, 77, 1061-1072.

Ogilvie, D. M., Stone, P. J., & Shneidman, E. S. (1965). Some characteristics of genuine versus simulated suicide notes. *Bulletin of Suicidology*, March, 27-32.

Osgood, C., & Walker, E. G. (1959). Motivation and language behavior. *Journal of Abnormal & Social Psychology*, 59, 58-67.

Park, B. C. B. (2004). Sociopolitical contexts of self-immolations in Vietnam and South Korea. *Archives of Suicide Research*, 8, 81-97.

Park, B. C. B., & Lester, D. (2009). Protest suicide. *Perceptual & Motor Skills*, 109, 917-920.

Pavese, C. (1952). *Il mestiere di vivere* Turin, Italy: Einaudi

Pavese, C. (1961). *The burning brand*. New York: Walker.

Peck, D. L. (1988-1989). Evaluation of a suicide diary. *Omega*, 19, 293-309.

Pennebaker, J. W. (1997). Writing about emotional experiences as a therapeutic process. *Psychological Science*, 8, 162-166.

Pennebaker, J. W., Francis, M. E., & Booth, R. J. (2001) *Linguistic inquiry and word count*. Mahwah, NJ: Erlbaum.

Pennebaker, J. W., & Stone, L. D. (2004). What was she trying to say? In D. Lester (Ed.) *Katie's diary*, pp. 55-79. New York: Brunner-Routledge.

Piaget, J. (1926). *The language and thought of the child*. New York: Harcourt, Brace & World.

Piotrowski, Z. A. (1974). *Perceptanalysis*. Philadelphia: privately published.

Pipher, M. (1994). *Reviving Ophelia*. New York: G. P. Putnam.

Plath, S. (1981) *The collected poems*. New York: Harper & Row.

Plath, S. (2000). *The unabridged journals of Sylvia Plath*. New York: Anchor Books.

Ramirez-Esparza, N., Pennebaker, J. W., Garcia, F. A., & Suria, R. (2007). [The psychology of word use.] *Revista Mexicana de Psicologia*, 24, 85-99. [In Spanish]

Rogan, R. G. (2009). Linguistic indicators of suicidality in crisis negotiations. *Journal of Police Crisis Negotiations*, 9, 34-54.

Rogers, C. R. (1961). The loneliness of contemporary man as seen in the case of Ellen West. *Annals of Psychotherapy*, 2, 94-101.

Rogers, J. R. (2001). Theoretical grounding: the "missing link" in suicide research. *Journal of Counseling & Development*, 79, 16-25.

Rogers, J. R., Bromley, J. L., McNally, C. J., & Lester, D. (2007). Content analysis of suicide notes as a test of the motivational component of the existential-constructivist model of suicide. *Journal of Counseling & Development*, 85, 182-188.

Rudestam, K. E. (1977). Physical and psychological responses to suicide in the family. *Journal of Consulting & Clinical Psychology*, 45, 162-170.

Rudestam, K. E. (1990). Survivors of suicide. In D. Lester (Ed.), *Current issues in suicide research*. Philadelphia, PA: Charles Press.

Runeson, B., & Asberg, M. (2003). Family history of suicide among suicide victims. *American Journal of Psychiatry*, 160, 1525-1526.

Sakamoto, S. (1998). The preoccupation scale. *Journal of Clinical Psychology*, 54, 645-654.

Sands, B. (1998). *Writings from prison*. Dublin, Ireland: Mercier Press.

Seiden, R., & Tauber, R. (1970). Pseudocides versus suicides. In *Proceedings of the 5th International Congress for Suicide Prevention*, pp. 219-223. Vienna, Austria: International Association for Suicide Prevention.

Shakespeare, W. (1969). *William Shakespeare: The complete works*. Ed. by A. Harbage. London, UK: Penguin.

Sheskin, A., & Wallace, S. E. (1976). Differing bereavements. *Omega*, 7, 229-242.

Shneidman, E. S. (1982). The suicidal logic of Cesare Pavese. *Journal of the American Academy of Psychoanalysis*, 10, 547-563.

Shneidman, E. S. (1994). The Inman diary. In A. A. Leenaars, J. T. Maltsberger & R. A. Neimeyer (Eds.) *Treatment of suicidal people*, pp. 3-15. Washington, DC: Taylor & Francis.

Shneidman, E .S. (1996). *The suicidal mind.* New York: Oxford University Press.

Shneidman, E. S., & Farberow, N. L. (1957a). The logic of suicide. In E. S. Shneidman & N. L. Farberow (Eds.) *Clues to suicide*, pp. 31-40. New York: McGraw-Hill.

Shneidman, E. S., & Farberow, N. L. (1957b). (Eds.) *Clues to suicide*. New York: McGraw-Hill.

Shneidman, E. S., & Farberow, N. L. (1957c). Some comparisons between genuine and simulated suicide notes in terms of Mowrer's concepts of discomfort and relief. *Journal of General Psychology*, 56, 251-256.

Silverman, M. A., & Will, N. P. (1986). Sylvia Plath and the failure of emotional self-repair through poetry. *Psychoanalytic Quarterly*, 55: 99-129.

Spiegel, D., & Neuringer, C. (1963). Role of dread in suicidal behavior. *Journal of Abnormal & Social Psychology*, 66, 507-511.

Srabstein, J. (2008). Bullying: a global public health risk. *International Journal of Adolescent Medicine & Health*, 20, 99-100.

Stack, S., Lester, D., & Rosenberg, J. S. (2012). Music and suicidality. *Suicide & Life-Threatening Behavior*, 42, 654-671.

Stack, S., & Wasserman, I. (2007). Economic strain and suicide risk: a qualitative analysis. *Suicide & Life-Threatening Behavior*, 37, 103-112.

Stefanone, M. A., & Jang, C. Y. (2008). Writing for friends and family. *Journal of Computer-Mediated Communication*, 13, 123-140.

Stirman, S. W., & Pennebaker, J. W. (2001). Word use in the poetry of suicidal and nonsuicidal poets. *Psychosomatic Medicine*, 63, 517-522.

Teasdale, S. (1938). *The collected poems of Sara Teasdale*. New York: Macmillan.

Tuckman, J., & Ziegler, R. (1966). Language usage and social maturity as related to suicide notes. *Journal of Social Psychology*, 68, 139-142.

Williams, F. M. (2007). The relationship among linguistic patterns, thwarted belongingness, perceived burdensomeness, and suicidal behavior. *Dissertation Abstracts International*, 67(8B), 4728.

Wolf, M., Horn, A., Mehl, M. R., Haug, S., Pennebaker, J., & Kordy, H. (2008). [Computer-aided quantitative text analysis] *Diagnostica*, 54(2), 85-98. (In German).

Yang, B., & Lester, D. (2011). The presentation of the self. *Suicidology Online*, 2, 75-79.

Zhang, J. (2005). [Conceptualizing a strain theory of suicide.] [*Chinese Mental Health Journal*], 19, 778-782. (In Chinese)

Zhang, J., & Lester, D. (2008). Psychological tensions found in suicide notes. *Archives of Suicide Research*, 12, 67-73.

Zijlstra, H., van Meerveld, T., van Middendorp, H., Pennebaker, J. W., & Geenen, R. (2004). [Dutch version of the Linguistic Inquiry Word Count (LIWC)] *Gedrag & Gezondheid*, 32, 272-281. (In Dutch)

Zipf, G. K. (1949). *Human behavior and the principle of least effort*. Cambridge, MA: Addison-Wesley.

Senior Author Index

W

Y

Z

Subject Index

T

V

W

Y

Bei Fragen zur Produktsicherheit wenden Sie sich bitte an:
If you have any questions regarding product safety,
please contact:

Walter de Gruyter GmbH
Genthiner Straße 13
10785 Berlin
productsafety@degruyterbrill.com